Praise for *The Pou*

WENDELL POTTER

The Power of Honest Medicine: LDN, an Inexpensive Alternative to the Costly, Toxic Medications Doctors Prescribe for Autoimmune and Other Diseases is a revealing look at the contradictions of our dysfunctional health care system—a system that often ignores potential benefits of low-risk, low-cost medications primarily because they lack sufficient profit potential for big pharmaceutical companies.

Julia Schopick presents the stories of a diverse group of patients with conditions that appeared hopeless for years but who persisted in finding solutions. This book is a vital resource for patients who want to become the authors of their own health.

Wendell Potter
Founder of Tarbell.org
Author:
—*Deadly Spin: An Insurance Company Insider Speaks Out on How Corporate PR Is Killing Health Care and Deceiving Americans*
—*Nation on the Take: How Big Money Corrupts Our Democracy and What We Can Do About It*

WAYNE JONAS, MD

Julia Schopick has shown again, like in her first book, *Honest Medicine*, that she is a skilled medical detective, finding pioneers and treatments that heal. If you have an autoimmune disease, read this book.

Wayne B. Jonas, MD
Executive Director, Samueli Health Programs
Former Director, NIH Office of Alternative Medicine
Author: *How Healing Works*

DAVID GLUCK, MD

The Power of Honest Medicine: LDN, an Inexpensive Alternative to the Costly, Toxic Medications Doctors Prescribe for Autoimmune and Other Diseases, by Julia Schopick (with Don Schwartz) is by far the clearest and finest book ever written for lay people regarding the effect of Low Dose Naltrexone on autoimmune diseases.

The book is filled with individual stories, presented in vivid detail, by people who went through heartbreaking difficulties for far too many years before they finally became aware of LDN and thus were often able "to get [their] lives back."

In addition, Schopick goes on to add a cornucopia of guidance, including advice on how to approach a physician when seeking a prescription for LDN, and the URLs for a host of online information such as: LDN websites in the USA and globally, disease-specific LDN groups, related forums, all past conferences, audios, videos, documentaries and books about LDN, the best known studies and clinical trials of LDN, sources for finding LDN-prescribing doctors, and lists of recommended LDN-compounding pharmacies.

I can't recommend this compelling and valuable book highly enough.

David Gluck, MD
Board-Certified Specialist in Internal Medicine and Preventive Medicine
Founder of the LDN website at http://www.LowDoseNaltrexone.org
Friend and Colleague of Dr. Bernard Bihari

VIRGINIA MCCULLOUGH

It was time for a comprehensive book that offers hope to patients suffering from complex and often misunderstood autoimmune diseases, and *The Power of Honest Medicine: LDN, an Inexpensive Alternative to the Costly, Toxic Medications Doctors Prescribe for Autoimmune and Other Diseases* is that book. If you or someone you love is coping with an autoimmune disease, you will want to read *The Power of Honest Medicine*. Written by Julia Schopick, author of *Honest Medicine*, this book meets a growing demand for up-to-date information about LDN, a safe and effective treatment for many conditions, including those falling under the umbrella term, autoimmune diseases.

Patients seeking therapies that differ from the mainstream treatment protocols for autoimmune disease often feel as if they live in two worlds simultaneously. And it isn't always easy to navigate from one to the other. In *The Power of Honest Medicine*, Schopick presents the stories of people who have been through the often long and grueling process of diagnoses and treatment for one of the 100+ autoimmune diseases. In their own words, these patients talk about their experiences with mainstream treatments and life before and after LDN. These patients had the tenacity and courage to look for effective treatments that didn't cause unpredictable and often dangerous side effects—and financial devastation due to their cost. Now they offer their stories to others.

In addition, Schopick provides information about ways to locate the treatment for those still seeking relief. I consider this an essential resource to help spread the word about the potential of LDN and the results it can produce for patients. I highly recommend it.

Virginia McCullough
Co-author: *The Oxygen Revolution*,
written with Paul Harch, MD, a pioneer in hyperbaric medicine

JACOB TEITELBAUM, MD

In a healthcare system where slick advertising masquerading as science has won out over truth in health education, it is a breath of fresh air to get honesty in medicine. This outstanding book by Julia Schopick and Don Schwartz discusses one of the most important medical discoveries of our time for addressing the modern epidemic of immune illness.

But you won't hear about this incredible research and treatment tool from your physician, because they won't hear about it from the drug companies. Why? Because it costs less than a dollar a day instead of $40,000 a year like most new immune drugs. So, nobody is paying to get the doctors this information. But here it is!

Got fibromyalgia, chronic pain, cancer, or an autoimmune illness such as Hashimoto's, Crohn's or rheumatoid arthritis? READ THIS BOOK. It can give you back your life!

Jacob Teitelbaum, MD
Physician
Creator of the popular free *"Cures A-Z"* phone app
Author:
—*From Fatigued to Fantastic*
—*The Fatigue and Fibromyalgia Solution*
—*Diabetes is Optional: Hintonia: The Natural Way to Control Type 2 Diabetes*

RONALD HOFFMAN, MD

I have treated patients in my practice with Low Dose Naltrexone for 30 years, and am happy that it is now soaring in popularity as a versatile tool in the armamentarium of innovative physicians. LDN occupies a unique place among medications because it leverages the body's own defenses to address a multitude of conditions—including but not limited to those conditions profiled in this book.

Julia Schopick does us a great service by breaking down the research, spiked with compelling patient success stories. I highly recommend this book!

Ronald Hoffman, MD
Founder, Hoffman Center
Author of 8 books, including:
—*How to Talk with Your Doctor*
—*Intelligent Medicine*
Host, "The Intelligent Medicine Podcast" (formerly "Health Talk")
Past President, American College for Advancement in Medicine (ACAM)
Board of Directors, Alliance for Natural Health (ANH)

BURT BERKSON, MD, MS, PhD

The Power of Honest Medicine: LDN, an Inexpensive Alternative to the Costly, Toxic Medications Doctors Prescribe for Autoimmune and Other Diseases is an intelligent tour through the science and day-to-day use of Low Dose Naltrexone by doctors and patients.

Well-respected author Julia Schopick describes an effective way to control several examples of autoimmune disease with the use of LDN in this well-written book. Through personal stories by patients and effective explanations by the author on the use of this amazing agent, I found this book easy and captivating to read.

Naltrexone was first approved in the 1980s as a prescription drug to reverse the effects of opiate poisoning. Low Dose Naltrexone is a very low dose of naltrexone and has been found to be effective in treating several diseases including systemic lupus erythematosus, rheumatoid arthritis, Crohn's disease, Parkinson's disease, certain cancers, etc.

I first learned about LDN about 20 years ago when a man presented to my clinic, using a walker, and who appeared very ill. He told me that he had rheumatoid arthritis and prostate cancer metastasized to his bones. He said that an oncologist at a well-respected cancer hospital in Texas told him that there was no effective treatment for his disease and that he should receive palliative therapy at a Hospice.

The man asked me if I would prescribe some narcotic tablets to help him with his pain, so he could get his wife with senile dementia admitted to a nursing home. Then he asked me if I had ever heard of Dr. Bihari in New York. I answered no. He told me that he had heard that Bihari was effectively treating metastatic cancer *and* autoimmune disease.

I advised him to go see Dr. Bihari. Maybe he could help him. He answered that Dr. Bihari was just in a little office. "If he was any good wouldn't he be associated with a large medical center?" I answered that if he could cure cancer, he might put a large cancer clinic out of business since they treat cancer and do not often cure cancer.

I did not see the gentleman for three years. I thought he had died. Then one day he appeared in our clinic complaining of a sinus infection. The man looked healthy and was standing straight and did not have the use of his walker. He told me that he saw Dr. Bihari and that his rheumatoid arthritis and prostate cancer became under control with a drug, that at that time cost only $15 a month: LDN.

I was very skeptical, but curious, and prescribed it to myself and several patients. It had no side effects and helped me sleep comfortably. Many of my patients reversed their lupus, dermatomyositis, autoimmune hepatitis, rheumatoid arthritis, and other autoimmune diseases with LDN.

Then I started prescribing it for cancer with the addition of intravenous alpha lipoic acid and observed the same remarkable results with several stage 4 cancer patients. Check "Berkson BM" in Google Scholar or PubMed, and Google "Berkson, National Cancer Institute." You will find some very amazing information there.

My colleagues and I published the first peer-reviewed publications on the reversal of stage four cancers in patients using LDN plus alpha lipoic acid.

In this exceptionally good book, Ms. Schopick describes the remarkable results people with autoimmune disease are having using LDN and the problems that many patients have persuading their doctors to prescribe this efficacious agent. The book is logical and methodical and provides a plan for the use of LDN for several autoimmune illnesses.

I genuinely enjoyed reading this book, and I would recommend it to doctors, patients, and anyone who wants a good read about a drug that is effective and almost completely ignored by the medical establishment.

Burton M. Berkson, MD, MS, PhD
Founder, the Integrative Medical Center of New Mexico, Las Cruces
Adjunct Professor, Oklahoma State College of Medicine, Tulsa
Former Professor, Rutgers University, and Chicago State University
Author: *The Alpha Lipoic Acid Breakthrough*
Co-author:
—*Syndrome X* (the first book on metabolic syndrome)
—*All About the B Vitamins*
—*User's Guide to the B-Complex Vitamins*

NASHA WINTERS, ND

I first became familiar with LDN in 1996 during my medical student clinical rotation in an HIV/AIDS clinic in Phoenix, Arizona. It was then that I learned of the work of Dr. Bernard Bihari.

The results I began to see with this seemingly innocuous little pill still astound me today: dark moods lifting, unresponsive skin conditions resolving, CD4 counts rising while viral titers dropped, less acute infections, and autoimmune illnesses such as rheumatoid arthritis and Hashimoto's autoimmune thyroiditis going into remission. It just didn't seem possible. And now, 22 years later, I continue to recommend LDN to thousands of patients and mentor hundreds of clinicians on its use. I even use it for my own collection of health issues with great results.

The Power of Honest Medicine, by Julia Schopick (with Don Schwartz), is an important book. Built on the foundation created by others who came before, the book brings us a deeper understanding of this powerful off-label drug.

Thank you so much, Julia, for your unwavering passion and ability to share the story and spread the word once again! The collection of voices you have pulled together in this book will create a powerful ripple effect in patient care for years to come. This is a truly remarkable book. I highly recommend it!

Nasha Winters, ND, FABNO
Founder and CEO, Optimal Terrain Consulting,
Co-founder of Terrain10
Co-author of the bestselling book: *The Metabolic Approach to Cancer*

THE POWER OF HONEST MEDICINE

LDN, an Inexpensive Alternative to the Costly, Toxic Medications Doctors Prescribe for Autoimmune and Other Diseases

*Low Dose Naltrexone Success Stories
From Patients Around the World*

MS, Rheumatoid Arthritis, Crohn's, Parkinson's, Lupus, Hashimoto's, Fibromyalgia, and More

By **Julia Schopick**
with
Don Schwartz, PhD

The Power of Honest Medicine:
LDN, an Inexpensive Alternative to the Costly, Toxic Medications Doctors Prescribe for Autoimmune and Other Diseases

Low Dose Naltrexone Success Stories From Patients Around the World

Copyright © 2018 Julia Schopick and Don Schwartz, PhD. All rights reserved. Printed in the United States of America. Except as permitted under the United States Copyright Act of 1976, no part of this publication may be reproduced or distributed in any form or by any means, or stored in a data base or retrieval system, without prior written permission of the publisher.

ISBN: 978-0-9829690-3-8

The information provided in this book should not be construed as personal medical advice or instruction. No action should be taken based solely on the contents of this publication. Readers should consult appropriate health professionals on any matter relating to their health and well-being. The information and opinions provided here are believed to be accurate and sound, based on the best judgment available to the authors, but readers who fail to consult appropriate health authorities assume the risk of any injuries.

Published by:

Innovative Health Publishing
Oak Park, Illinois
www.HonestMedicine.com

Editor: Mary Shomon
Cover Design: George Foster, Foster Covers
Layout Design: William Groetzinger

Dedication

The Power of Honest Medicine
is gratefully dedicated to

My father, Dr. Lou Schopick
(December 21, 1907 – February 27, 1976)
who taught me to be wary of the
medical establishment

and to

My mother, Sonya Turitz Schopick
who taught me to be open to treatments the
medical establishment doesn't know about

and to

My husband, Tim Fisher
(March 13, 1949 – November 8, 2005)
who changed my life forever.

I will be forever grateful to all three.

"Until the day I die, I will not stop fighting until this drug has gained respectability and acceptance in the medical community."

—Bernard Bihari, MD

Table of Contents

Acknowledgments
    Julia Schopick xv
    Don Schwartz xix

Introduction 1

Foreword 11

SECTION I: UNDERSTANDING LDN AND AUTOIMMUNITY 15
    Chapter 1: The LDN Story 17
    Chapter 2: Autoimmune Diseases 27

SECTION II: THE LDN HEROES 45
    Chapter 3: Fritz Bell (GoodShape.net) 47
    Chapter 4: Christina White (Brewer Science Library), the First Journalist to Write About LDN 57
    Chapter 5: How Frank Melhus Found Healing with Low Dose Naltrexone and Shared It with the World. 67
    Chapter 6: How Suffering with MS Turned Linda Elsegood into an LDN Hero: A Tribute to Persistence 79

SECTION III: THE STORIES. 93
    Introduction to the LDN Stories 95

Contributors with One Disease
    Chapter 7: Lad Jelen, Crohn's Disease 99
    Chapter 8: Maija Haavisto, Finland, Chronic Fatigue Syndrome/Myalgic Encephalomyelitis 107
    Chapter 9: John O'Connell, Hashimoto's Thyroiditis . . . 119

Chapter 10: May-Britt Hansen, Netherlands,
Hailey-Hailey Disease 127

Chapter 11: Andrea Schwung, Germany,
Multiple Sclerosis 135

Chapter 12: Emiliano Marchi, Italy,
Multiple Sclerosis 139

Chapter 13: Lexie Lindstrom, Parkinson's Disease 145

Chapter 14: Maureen Mirand, Rheumatoid Arthritis ... 159

Contributors with Multiple Conditions

Chapter 15: Monica Hovden, Norway,
Crohn's Disease and Fibromyalgia 171

Chapter 16: Renée Foster, Fibromyalgia and
Chronic Fatigue Syndrome 177

Chapter 17: Katrien Devriesere, Belgium,
Myalgic Encephalomyelitis/Chronic Fatigue
Syndrome, and Fibromyalgia 185

Chapter 18: Darlene Nichols, Lupus and
Myasthenia Gravis 193

Chapter 19: Kathy Shew, Psoriasis and
Multiple Sclerosis 203

Chapter 20: Margaret Schooling, France,
Rheumatoid Arthritis, a Blood Disorder,
a Tumor, and an Eye Problem 211

GOING FORWARD 219

Chapter 21: How to Convince Your Doctor to
Prescribe LDN for You 221

Afterword: The Media—For Good, and Not so Good... 229

APPENDICES

Appendix A: LDN Resources 239
    Websites—General. 239
    LDN Websites from Around the World 241
    Facebook Groups 242
    Other LDN Forums, Including Yahoo Groups 246
    LDN Conferences: 2005-2008. 247
    LDN Conferences: 2009-2019. 249
    Audios and Videos 252
    Books About LDN. 252
    Books that Contain Information About LDN 254
    LDN Documentaries 255
    LDN Prescribing Doctors. 256
    Compounding Pharmacies 256
    LDN Studies 257
    Other Studies and Trials. 258
    Postscript: Update 259
    Easy Access to this Book's Hyperlinks. 260

Appendix B: About the Authors. 261
    Julia Schopick 261
    Don Schwartz 262

Endnotes. 265

Acknowledgments

Julia Schopick

I want to first thank Don Schwartz, without whom this book would not have seen the light of day.

I started to write *The Power of Honest Medicine: LDN, an Inexpensive Alternative to the Costly, Toxic Medications Doctors Prescribe for Autoimmune and Other Diseases* in 2013, shortly after my first book, *Honest Medicine*, was published. The LDN patient stories featured there were all about multiple sclerosis. As I started appearing as a guest on talk shows, it became obvious that people with many other autoimmune conditions were interested in this treatment—and were having excellent results with it.

Slowly, I began interviewing these people, with the goal of turning their stories into a book.

But that didn't happen so quickly. After interviewing several, and having their interviews transcribed and edited into chapter form, I put the idea aside.

Then I met Don. When I told him about this book, which I had virtually abandoned, he said, "You can't do that! LDN is too important a treatment. You've got to publish this book!" When I demurred, he said he'd be happy to work on it with me.

And so he did. He went over every chapter with me, offering his edits and his suggestions. Whenever I'd get discouraged, Don would prop me up. And his excitement finally became contagious.

Although Don is my co-author, he pointed out that writing the book with a "we" voice might be confusing to readers, so he insisted that we write the book in my voice. That's what we did.

After Don, I want to thank those who have contributed their experiences to this book, starting with Jackie Young Bihari, the widow of Dr. Bernard Bihari, without whom there would have been no Low Dose Naltrexone. Throughout the years, Jackie has been supportive of my work, including my book *Honest Medicine* (which she has shared with scores of people!), and of this new book. She contributed the foreword.

I also want to thank the LDN Heroes featured here: Fritz Bell, creator of the early website, goodshape.net, devoted to spreading the word about LDN; Frank Melhus, producer of the Norwegian documentary about LDN; Christina White, the first journalist to write about LDN; and Linda Elsegood, whose non-profit organization and website, LDNResearchTrust.org, has done so much to spread the word about LDN. The devotion of these heroes has fostered LDN's growth into what I am fond of referring to as a *cause célèbre*. My sincere thanks to each of you for contributing your powerful stories to this book.

And of course, thanks to the patients whose stories are here: Maija Haavisto, John O'Connell, May-Britt Hansen, Andrea Schwung, Emiliano Marchi, Lexie Lindstrom, Maureen Mirand, Monica Hovden, Renée Foster, Katrien Devriesere, Darlene Nichols, Kathy Shew, Margaret Schooling, and the late Lad Jelen. Each of you spent hours with me, fine-tuning your chapters—some on the phone, others via email, and still others (those of you in Europe) on Skype. Without your stories, there would be no book.

I would also like to thank two people who did not provide their own stories, but who helped me in other ways. First, Manda-Marieke Schuurer, administrator of the Dutch/Belgium LDN Facebook group, who not only translated Katrien Devriesere's chapter but also participated in Skype conversations with us to fine-tune it. Second, Isabella Bresci, who is working so diligently to get both *Honest Medicine*, and now, *The Power of Honest Medicine*, published in Italy in Italian. Thanks to both of you!

Thanks, too, to those people who provided me with interviews, but whose stories, for various reasons, were not included: Michelle Anderson Jones, Terry Paulding, Allan Sustare, Cindy Surval, Melissa Bowles, and Isabella Perennis.

Thanks to my friends: Virginia McCullough, who initially worked with me on this book, and contributed heavily to the chapter about autoimmune diseases. We have been friends and colleagues for over 30 years. Also, Rose Nelson, who provided emotional support throughout the writing process; Beth Ryza and Harry Steckman; Pam Ransom; Ann McCabe; Philippa Norman; Michelle Gerencser; and Kathy and Ned Bezinovich. Your friendship throughout the years has meant so much to me!

And thanks to two new friends who provided invaluable counsel and support: Paul Berlanga, for going through the manuscript and sharing his time and brilliance with me. Paul, your valuable critique helped to make this book what it is. I'll be forever grateful to you. And Fred Reklau, who has the sharpest eyes. Fred caught almost every typo!

And I can't forget Peter de Zordo, who translated Emiliano Marchi's original chapter from the Italian. *Grazie, mio caro amico!*

There are two special friends I'd like to thank: Dr. Burt Berkson and Mary Jo Bean. I met both through the writing of *Honest Medicine*, and they have both become trusted, very close, friends. Our many-hour phone conversations have meant the world to me. I love you both.

And I can't forget these five people: my business coach, Betty Rockendorf, whose faith in me throughout the writing process has kept me going; Mary Shomon, for your friendship, your sharp eyes, your edits, and your excellent suggestions; Paula Allen, for transcribing the Skype interviews with my European contributors; Cathy Lewis, for your public relations support throughout the years; and Fritz Bell, whom I already mentioned as one of the book's LDN Heroes, for being such an enthusiastic friend and cheerleader!

And a hearty thanks to all my Facebook friends and followers. There are literally thousands of you. I can't name all of you here, but you know who you are. Your acceptance of my work, and your support throughout the years, have meant the world to me.

And you, George Foster, for your book covers, both for *Honest Medicine* and *The Power of Honest Medicine*. What would I ever do without you? You have proven to me—twice—that you CAN tell a book by its cover. Bless your heart!

And Chuck Poch, because without your technological brilliance, I would have been dead in the water many years ago.

Lastly, I want to thank my parents, to whom this book is dedicated. My dad, Dr. Lou Schopick, taught me to use my head and NOT follow everything doctors told me. His words of foreboding ring in my ears every day: "If a doctor tells you he knows all the answers, run like hell!" Thanks, Dad!

And to my Mom, Sonya Schopick, whose own mother, my Grandma Julia, went to Germany for an experimental treatment in 1928, after being told by Dr. Charles Mayo that she had only six months to live. That experimental treatment—unavailable at the time in the US—allowed my grandmother to live eleven more years, leaving my Mom without a mother at the age of 22, rather than age 11. Largely because of this experience, Mom has been a champion of my point of view, and of my efforts, from the very beginning. She was, in fact, the primary editor and typo-catcher *par excellence* of *Honest Medicine*. As I write this book, Mom is in hospice. How I wish she were able to catch typos for this book. So, if there are any, it's her fault!

And I couldn't end these acknowledgments without giving a huge thanks to my late husband, Tim Fisher. It was my experience of being Tim's wife, caregiver, and advocate during the fifteen years after his diagnosis with a brain tumor that turned me into an advocate for others, as well as the author of both *Honest Medicine* and *The Power of Honest Medicine*. I wish we didn't have to go through that experience—and I dearly wish Tim were still here with me. But he provided the inspiration which has guided all of my efforts for so many years.

Don Schwartz

First and foremost, gratitude to the amazing Julia Schopick for this opportunity to support her crucial contribution to our world. Thanks to Julia, I take Low Dose Naltrexone every day and anticipate doing so the rest of my life. I could not have participated in the creation of this book without the generous support of Peter de Zordo and David Hakim. And, I would not have met Julia had it not been for our mutual Facebook friend, Paul Meilleur.

Introduction

I am delighted to introduce *The Power of Honest Medicine: LDN, an Inexpensive Alternative to the Costly, Toxic Medications Doctors Prescribe for Autoimmune and Other Diseases,* the second book in my "Honest Medicine" series. *Honest Medicine,* which was published in 2011, featured four treatments for life-threatening diseases: Silverlon for non-healing wounds; intravenous alpha lipoic acid for terminal liver disease; the Ketogenic Diet for childhood epilepsy; and Low Dose Naltrexone (LDN) for autoimmune diseases and some cancers.

All four were enormously valuable treatments in that they were—as the book's subtitle asserted—"effective, time-tested, inexpensive," and helped people with life-threatening diseases. I set the bar extremely high for each of the four featured treatments. For instance, to fit the criterion of "time-tested," the treatments had to have been helping people for at least 25 years. This might seem arbitrary, but as many of you know, physicians often deny the effectiveness of a treatment by claiming that the evidence is insufficient and that reports of its effectiveness are merely "anecdotal." However, if a treatment has been successfully used for 25 or more years—as is the case with each of the treatments in *Honest Medicine*—it's more difficult to dismiss positive results as merely isolated patient stories.

"Inexpensive" was a criterion added for a personal reason. When my husband Tim was ill with a brain tumor, we worked hard to extend the quality of his life and the years we'd have together. The bottom line: We went broke, paying out of pocket for treatments not covered by insurance. Some of the treatments helped him; others did not. But together, they consumed vast amounts of money.

By introducing treatments that are more effective *and* less expensive than the conventional treatments most doctors recommend, *Honest Medicine* helped people avoid the soul-crushing experience of going broke while taking care of themselves and their loved ones.

The severity of the conditions treated was also a factor. I focused on treatments for serious, debilitating, and life-threatening conditions like non-healing wounds, terminal liver disease, intractable epilepsy, and autoimmune diseases such as multiple sclerosis (MS), lupus, rheumatoid arthritis (RA), and Crohn's disease.

I was tireless in my efforts to get the word out about these treatments and found that radio talk shows were an effective way to reach the public. In the seven years since *Honest Medicine's* publication, I have appeared on several hundred shows, and am often invited back. Each time I did a show, I heard from many people desperate for more information about the treatments featured in the book.

Of the four, Low Dose Naltrexone (LDN) consistently generated the most interest and received the largest response from listeners. Interviewers and callers clamored for more information about this low-cost, off-label[1] treatment for various autoimmune diseases. After each interview, I'd get an influx of emails and calls about LDN, mostly from people who had been diagnosed with an autoimmune disease such as MS, Crohn's disease, or fibromyalgia—or other conditions I'd mentioned on a particular program.

After my first appearance on *Coast to Coast AM,* one of the most popular radio call-in shows in the country, my book shot up to number 49 on the Amazon bestseller list, and I received more than 400 emails and more than 50 phone calls. My second appearance on this show generated a similar response. *Almost all the listeners asked about LDN.* They weren't just curious about it. They were angry that their doctors had never told them about it, and they wanted my help in convincing their doctors to prescribe LDN for them.

I counseled hundreds of people around the world about how to work with their doctors to get LDN and followed up to hear their experiences. I also heard from patients who were already enjoying the remarkable benefits of this drug for their autoimmune conditions. Over time, I amassed a great deal of information, including small studies and patient successes. I refer to the latter as "patient-based evidence." I shared this information with listeners who contacted me so that they, in turn, could give it to their doctors. If the information I sent them didn't convince their doctors, they wrote back, asking me for help finding a doctor who *would* prescribe LDN for them. Thanks to a list of prescribing doctors put together by LDN patient advocate Crystal Nason, I was able to help. It was a full-time job answering the requests, and there were so many inquiries that I started conducting teleseminars[2] and coaching sessions[3] to help patients convince their doctors to prescribe LDN. I share these strategies in Chapter 21.

I also became active on Facebook, where I found groups devoted to sharing information about LDN. There were several groups for patients with autoimmune diseases in general, as well as groups for patients with specific conditions, including Hashimoto's thyroiditis, rheumatoid arthritis, Crohn's disease and irritable bowel syndrome, fibromyalgia, chronic fatigue syndrome, etc. I joined and became active in many of these groups, as well as in some in other countries, including Norway, the Netherlands, Germany, France, Italy, Spain, Poland, Turkey, and Brazil. For the international groups, I used Google Translate to participate in discussions. There are also several websites, both in the US and abroad, devoted to spreading the word about LDN. These groups and websites are listed in the Appendix.

In 2013, Frank Melhus, a producer at TV2 in Norway, aired a documentary devoted to Low Dose Naltrexone, as part of the station's *Vårt Lille Land* ("Our Small Country") series.[4] The numbers of people using LDN in Norway soon skyrocketed from 200 to 300, to 15,000. [Author's Note: There is now a version of the documentary on YouTube with English subtitles, and versions with Italian, French and German subtitles are in the works.] Worldwide interest in LDN was growing. Along the way, *Honest Medicine* was translated and published in Poland and the Netherlands; a Spanish edition is now available. Of the four treatments, LDN is of greatest interest to international publishers.

Because of this response, I am devoting this second book entirely to LDN. There is another important reason. According to the American Autoimmune Related Diseases Association (AARDA),[5] autoimmune diseases are on the rise. At last count, over 100 different diseases categorized as autoimmune have been identified—and they affect a staggering number of people in the US, as well as internationally. Some people are affected by more than one autoimmune disease. More people in the US are affected by autoimmune diseases than by cancer, and they are among the top ten causes of death in the US. Treatment for autoimmune diseases is also extremely costly. According to one estimate, over $100 billion is spent annually on autoimmune disease. This is likely an underestimate, considering that it's estimated that it costs between $51.8 and $70.6 billion annually to treat just seven, namely Crohn's disease, ulcerative colitis, lupus, MS, rheumatoid arthritis, psoriasis, and scleroderma.

There is evidence that LDN is a groundbreaking treatment for autoimmune diseases, helping some patients with these diseases to achieve remission. In other cases, it can slow or stop the progression of their disease. In most cases, patients experience a life-changing relief of symptoms. LDN is safe, inexpensive, non-toxic, virtually free of side effects (the most common being "vivid dreams"), and often dramatically effective. The challenge: LDN remains relatively unknown to many doctors and patients.

This has to change.

In my opinion, LDN is one of the most important medical discoveries of the twentieth century. Hundreds of doctors who prescribe it, and thousands of patients who use it, agree. LDN—which works for so many conditions—is also the cheapest and most versatile of the treatments I have encountered.

When people first hear about LDN for autoimmune diseases, many are puzzled. They may be familiar with the drug naltrexone and know that it is a drug typically used to treat addictions. Naltrexone is a narcotic blocker approved by the FDA in the mid-1980s for people with drug addiction. In the mid-1990s, naltrexone was also approved for alcohol addiction. Naltrexone is typically prescribed at doses starting at 50 mg or more for people with drug addiction. It has been "off-patent" for many years, meaning that there is no "branded" naltrexone that is manufactured and marketed by a drug company. Generic naltrexone tablets cost little to produce and are typically inexpensive.

In studying the use of naltrexone for addictions, Harvard-educated neurologist-psychiatrist Bernard Bihari, MD discovered and then pioneered the use of naltrexone in very low doses—typically less than 5 mg per day—for autoimmune diseases. Dr. Bihari reported excellent results with MS, , Crohn's disease, RA, lupus, and many other conditions, including AIDS.[6]

Since Dr. Bihari introduced LDN therapy, thousands of patients with serious, debilitating conditions have experienced tremendous relief using LDN. In the beginning, and even today, some patients purchase generic 50 mg naltrexone tablets and make their own LDN. There are also pharmacists in the US who have the expertise to compound LDN correctly.[7] Because of patient demand, the number of pharmacists worldwide who compound LDN is growing daily.

Because there is minimal profit in LDN, it has not been the subject of costly, large-scale FDA trials. But smaller studies conducted at leading institutions have been published in prominent publications and are backing up the reports of patient success. There were three studies on LDN for Crohn's disease conducted at Penn State;[8][9][10] three studies conducted at Stanford University using LDN for fibromyalgia;[11][12][13] one for multiple sclerosis at the University of California at San Francisco;[14] and yet another for multiple sclerosis in Milan, Italy.[15] Recently, there have been two studies for Hailey-Hailey disease (HHD),[16][17] one of which was performed at Emory University in Atlanta. More small studies are being conducted at the time of this writing.

Spreading the Word

I feel it is crucial to significantly expand LDN awareness. While a handful of doctors in the US and abroad are passionate about LDN, most doctors still reflexively prescribe the more toxic, side-effect-laden, expensive drugs—many of which don't work particularly well for their patients. To make matters worse, even when presented with compelling information, many doctors refuse outright to prescribe LDN.

Currently, people with autoimmune disorders who research their conditions can find out about LDN on the Internet. Those who discover LDN often do so after having already been prescribed—and been disappointed or even harmed by—more toxic drugs. Thankfully, finding information about LDN online is becoming easier, with several US and international LDN websites, as well as forums and chat groups devoted to discussions about LDN.

You will find information about these websites, chat groups and forums in the Appendix.

At the same time, more doctors and health care providers are becoming aware of and showing interest in LDN. They are attending and speaking at conferences that are being held to educate doctors and patients about this treatment. So far, there have been more than a dozen LDN conferences in the US and Europe,[18] [19] almost every year since 2005.

The LDN conferences have taken place in large part thanks to the hard work and dedication of two people: David Gluck, MD, Dr. Bihari's colleague and the creator of one of the most respected LDN websites;[20] and Linda Elsegood, creator of another, equally respected LDN site.[21] Through Linda's not-for-profit organization and website, the LDN Research Trust, she has also interviewed hundreds of doctors, patients and compounding pharmacists about their successes with LDN.[22] These video interviews are featured on Vimeo.[23] Thanks to Linda, you can also learn about other websites and Facebook groups throughout the world that spread the word about LDN.[24] She also has an online radio show dedicated to increasing LDN awareness.

A few years ago, as part of my commitment to LDN awareness, I began conducting LDN teleseminars,[25] to help patients become informed about LDN and provide them with enough convincing information to share with their doctors. I also conduct personal and group coaching sessions[26] for patients who want more individualized attention. These proactive patients report that when they are prepared with knowledge, printed information, and effective communications tactics, their doctors respond better to their requests for LDN prescriptions.

In Chapter 21, I share this information with you.

Although Dr. Bihari died in May of 2010, his legacy continues. Thanks to Dr. Bihari's perseverance for over a quarter of a century, and his success with treating patients throughout those years, more physicians around the world are now using LDN to treat autoimmune and other diseases. But let's be clear: It's the proverbial drop in the bucket. Millions of people continue to suffer from autoimmune diseases, and most of them—as well as their health care providers—are unaware of LDN's potential to alter the course of their illness and improve their health.

This book is devoted to changing that.

As you read, you will better understand the concept of autoimmunity, as well as key information about LDN itself: how it works and why it is so important. You will also read the testimonies of patients from the US and around the world whose autoimmune conditions have been helped with LDN—conditions including lupus, myasthenia gravis, Hashimoto's thyroiditis, rheumatoid arthritis, fibromyalgia, Crohn's disease, chronic fatigue syndrome, and Parkinson's disease.

You'll meet four people I consider to be LDN Heroes: 1) Christina White, the first person we know of to write about LDN—for the Brewer Science Library's newsletter; 2) Fritz Bell, whose successful use of LDN for his wife Polly's MS led him to help scores of patients to get LDN; 3) the previously mentioned Frank Melhus, whose LDN documentary for Norwegian television led to a groundswell of interest in and use of LDN in Norway and, because of its presence on the Internet, around the world; and 4) Linda Elsegood who, through her United Kingdom charity, the LDN Research Trust, has done so much to spread the word about LDN, holding almost-yearly conferences and interviewing over 700 (so far) LDN advocates worldwide.

The patients featured in this book have had impressive results taking LDN for a number of conditions. For instance, Lexie Lindstrom found that most of her Parkinson's disease symptoms have nearly disappeared. She now spends much of her time helping other Parkinson's patients learn about and obtain LDN. She has appeared numerous times on Dr. Robert Rodgers' Parkinson's Recovery radio program, advocating for LDN, and has invited me to be a guest with her on the show several times.[27] [28] [29] [30]

Darlene Nichols suffered from two autoimmune diseases: lupus and myasthenia gravis. With LDN, which she found 20 years after her lupus diagnosis and 34 years after the onset of her symptoms, the symptoms of both diseases have disappeared.

You'll also read about how the many surgeries Lad Jelen underwent for his Crohn's disease before he found LDN, caused him to have serious complications he would not have experienced if he had found LDN earlier—complications that probably led to his death. While we lost Lad in 2014, his widow Peggy told me that he was proud to be a part of this book. Thanks to her help, you will get to read Lad's story.

I invite you to share the life-changing information in this book with friends, family, and colleagues who could be helped by taking LDN. And please support the LDN Revolution by sharing the information—as well as this book—with doctors and healthcare professionals around the world.

Wishing you good health!

— **Julia Schopick**

Foreword

Jacqueline Young Bihari was LDN pioneer Dr. Bernard Bihari's partner for 21 years and worked with him in his medical practice as his assistant. Jackie Bihari was also the president of Dr. Bihari's Foundation for Integrative Research (FIR), a non-profit, 501(c)(3) foundation for the research and development of Low Dose Naltrexone and met-enkephalin (opioid growth factor/OGF) for the treatment of AIDS. Since his death, Jackie has continued to work tirelessly to further Dr. Bihari's mission to increase awareness and acceptance of LDN.

My introduction to Low Dose Naltrexone occurred when I first met my partner, Dr. Bernard Bihari, back in 1991, in his medical office on West 15th Street, in New York City.

Dr. Bihari was so excited when he introduced me to LDN and showed me how this remarkable drug was making such progress in boosting the immune system, helping so many of his HIV/AIDS patients increase their T-cells, and improve their blood work. It was also helping patients with numerous other autoimmune diseases.

Dr. Bihari would choose a particular patient at random, show me their chart, go over their most recent blood work, and show me how much their results had improved by just taking LDN 4.5 mg. Back then, the only drug to take was AZT. At high doses, AZT was so toxic that it killed many HIV/AIDS patients. LDN has very few side effects, the most common of which are vivid dreams and insomnia. In most cases, these side effects drop off with regular use.

Dr. Bihari soon found that not only was LDN effective for HIV/AIDS, but also for multiple sclerosis, Parkinson's disease, many cancers, chronic fatigue syndrome, rheumatoid arthritis, and many other autoimmune diseases.

Dr. Bihari had countless meetings with various pharmaceutical companies and hospital-based physicians. He would show them all of the test results he had compiled after hours and days of research. They would not accept or believe any of the dramatic improvements his patients experienced. Instead, they just shrugged it off to "whatever"—and out the door they went.

This went on for years—rejection after rejection—and they would come up with some ridiculous excuse not to believe in LDN. He was called a "witch doctor," "snake oil man," and "a joke,"—but he continued to hold his head high. All this rejection just gave Dr. Bihari an even greater incentive to work harder than ever, and he did—night and day. He hardly ever took a day off or went on a vacation.

In addition to this lack of interest from pharmaceutical companies and doctors, Dr. Bihari's research papers about LDN to treat autoimmune diseases were effectively censored by medicine's prestigious journals. He was able to get his medical articles published in these journals most of his professional life before he started working with LDN. And there was a brief period of openness to LDN—in the early 1980s when he began using LDN to treat AIDS patients. Then, his papers were accepted for publication by such prestigious journals as *The Lancet*, and he was invited to give oral presentations at AIDS conferences around the world. But, when he began writing about his work with LDN for multiple sclerosis, chronic fatigue syndrome, herpes, and other autoimmune diseases, none of these journals would accept his articles.

There were, however, a few publications—mostly local newsletters that physicians didn't read—that were an immense help: *Poz Magazine* (Sean Strub was the editor), *The Advocate*, Dr. Julian Whitaker's *Health and Healing Newsletter*, and *The Brewer Science*

Library Newsletter. But no major publication would touch it. We even contacted *The Oprah Show*, *60 Minutes*, the Elton John AIDS Foundation, and Montel Williams, who has MS—not even one reply.

Dr. Bihari was a fierce fighter, and he told me, "Until the day I die, I will not stop fighting until this drug has gained respectability and acceptance in the medical community."

As fate would have it, after Dr. Bihari's passing in 2010, several books—fifteen at last count—have been written about LDN and most of them are available on Amazon.com. A few of the titles are, of course, Julia Schopick's brilliant first book, *Honest Medicine*; *The LDN Book*, by Linda Elsegood; *Children with Starving Brains*, by Dr. Jaquelyn McCandless; *The Promise of Low Dose Naltrexone Therapy*, by Elaine Moore and Samantha Wilkinson; *Up the Creek with a Paddle*, by Mary Boyle Bradley; *Google LDN*, by Joseph Wouk; and *LDN for Parkinson's Disease*, by Marlene "Lexie" Lindstrom. Others are being written all the time.

There have been successful clinical trials in Africa and the US using LDN for various autoimmune diseases, and interest in LDN grows every day.

Although Dr. Bihari is no longer with us, his Low Dose Naltrexone is, and one day it is going to be available to the masses. Countless numbers of people will reap the benefits of his unending belief in his drug.

Dr. Bihari's story would make a remarkable film. He invented this drug by himself—no help from anyone—did his own testing and research for years at his own expense, and invested all of his own money. I am sure he is now watching all of this with a big "I told you so" to all of his detractors with a big smile on his face.

Thank you, Dr. Bihari, for this gift to the world.

— **Jacqueline Young Bihari**

SECTION I:

UNDERSTANDING LDN AND AUTOIMMUNITY

CHAPTER 1

The LDN Story

> *If everything has to be double-blinded, randomized, and evidence-based, where does that leave new ideas?*
> July 9, 2005, The Lancet[31]

To understand the history of how LDN came to be used as a treatment for autoimmune diseases, it's important to know something about *naltrexone*, the drug from which LDN is compounded. Approved at 50 mg by the US Food and Drug Administration (FDA) in 1984 as a treatment for opiate addiction, naltrexone stops the effects of these opiates by blocking the receptors for the opioid hormones—also known as endorphins—that the body naturally produces. In the mid-1990s, naltrexone was also approved by the FDA, again at 50 mg, to treat alcohol dependence. In many people, it significantly reduced their cravings for opioids and/or alcohol.

Unfortunately, as LDN pioneer Dr. Bernard Bihari pointed out,[32] high doses of naltrexone frequently proved to be intolerable and often toxic. He reported:

> I gave it to about two dozen heroin addicts who had recently stopped using heroin. None of them would stay on it. At the doses involved it caused anxiety, depression, irritability. They couldn't sleep, and even minor stresses that they could handle the day before, they couldn't cope with on days that they took naltrexone in the morning.

Despite these significant side effects at high doses, naltrexone is still marketed in Europe and the US for drug and alcohol addiction under the brand names Vivitrol, Revia, and Depade. And while naltrexone was approved at 50 mg, some doctors used and still use it at doses up to 300 mg.

The FDA approves many drugs for specific uses, but over time, these drugs turn out to be beneficial as treatments for other conditions. Prescribing a drug for a condition that hasn't been approved by the FDA is known as "off-label" use of that drug. Any doctor is legally able to prescribe any FDA-approved drug off label, and some specialists, including cardiologists and oncologists, are known to prescribe drugs off label more often than other specialists. Pharmaceutical manufacturers are, however, legally prohibited from marketing their drugs for any off-label uses.

When doctors do prescribe a drug for off-label use, they tend to prescribe that drug at the same dose approved for "on-label" use. In some cases, however, a substantial change to dosage can have a significant effect on how that drug performs, and what it achieves. This is the case with LDN.

In the introduction, I referred to Dr. Bernard Bihari as one of my heroes. As a neurologist and psychiatrist treating drug addiction in New York City, Dr. Bihari found that many of his patients also had HIV, the virus that often leads to AIDS. [Author's Note: At the time when Dr. Bihari was working with these patients, the disease was as-yet unnamed.] On a hunch, knowing that naltrexone raised endorphin levels and caused the immune system to act correctly, he tried prescribing very low doses, around 3 mg[33] to these patients, hoping it would positively affect their disease. He was significantly changing the dosage. As noted, naltrexone is typically prescribed at 50 mg or more—and used for an entirely different purpose and illness. Dr. Bihari saw such positive results among his patients with HIV that by the mid-1990s, he began prescribing LDN for cancer patients as well.

In a 2003 radio interview on public radio in New York with Dr. Kamau Kokayi,[34] Dr. Bihari stated that he had treated 420 cancer patients with LDN, and that, on average, cancer stopped growing in about two-thirds of the patients. For half of that group, after six to eight months, he said their cancer went on to slowly shrink and disappear entirely. These are impressive results!

Recently, there has been renewed interest in using LDN for cancer. Physicians/researchers in the UK at St. George's University have been using LDN in combination with chemotherapies and natural treatments such as vitamin D3 and have found that the combination has been very effective for cancer patients. The documentary, *The Game Changer: LDN & Cancer*, sharing the experience of these researchers, was produced by Linda Elsegood and the LDN Research Trust. It is online at https://vimeo.com/168562089.

Dr. Bihari also noted that many patients with autoimmune diseases often improved after taking LDN once daily at bedtime. He also saw that LDN didn't produce the troublesome side effects his addiction patients experienced at high doses. His patients reported significant relief of their symptoms, without the adverse effects of so many of the immune-suppressing medications doctors typically prescribed for autoimmune diseases. Word started to spread, and more people came to New York to consult with Dr. Bihari, so they could be treated with this drug, which many called a "miracle."

How LDN Works

When naltrexone is used off-label in such a dramatically reduced dosage, it profoundly changes the way the drug behaves in the body. Patients taking LDN for autoimmune diseases never refer to taking "naltrexone," because LDN and naltrexone are not interchangeable terms.

LDN boosts endorphin levels. You probably know that endorphins produce a sense of wellbeing similar to what is termed a "runner's high." Any strenuous exercise stimulates endorphin production as well. Endorphins, also part of the immune system, are among the chemicals that function as natural pain relievers. Dr. Bihari discovered that people with autoimmune diseases and cancers have lower endorphin levels. Since endorphins help the immune system work properly, this is the crucial dynamic that clarifies why LDN helps so many conditions.[35]

David Gluck MD, Dr. Bihari's colleague, and himself a devoted advocate of LDN, explains why he feels LDN is unique.

> LDN is a brand-new paradigm, a new way of thinking of treatment. Instead of the medication actually doing the work, LDN goes into the body and essentially tricks the body by forcing it to double and triple its output of endorphins and metenkephalin, also known as opioid growth factor (OGF). Those endorphins and metenkephalin, in turn, cause the immune system to strengthen.
>
> The moment the immune system is strengthened by LDN, it remembers that its first and most important job is to never attack itself. By taking LDN, the diseases stop progressing because the immune system now is strengthened, so it no longer attacks "self."
>
> I think that medicine has been waiting for a way to safely strengthen the immune system for all these years, and I think we've finally got it.

For a more detailed explanation of how LDN works, I recommend that you explore the resources at the LDN Research Trust.[36]

LDN also appears to benefit, with varying degrees of success, some conditions that don't yet fit under the rubric of autoimmune disease—conditions such as ALS (Lou Gehrig's disease) and Alzheimer's disease. And as you will see when you read May-Britt

Hansen's contribution, LDN also helps people with Hailey-Hailey disease, a genetic—rather than autoimmune—skin condition.

Taking LDN

Patients are most often advised to take LDN at bedtime. Some patients, however, such as Kathy Shew (Chapter 19), who experience sleep disturbances taking LDN at night, take it early in the day, and have good results. Taking LDN at night is still advised, because when the brain is at rest during sleep, LDN temporarily blocks endorphins from attaching to opioid receptors in the brain. The body responds to this signal by stepping up endorphin production. Thus, LDN works *with the body* to produce its own endorphins, which in turn stimulates activity among certain types of immune system cells, including natural killer (NK) cells, T and B cells, stem cells, and macrophages.

Equally important, LDN does not stimulate the immune system into over-activity, a key factor in autoimmune diseases. Instead, LDN helps modulate the inflammatory response and the production of neurotoxic chemicals in the brain.

You need a prescription to obtain LDN. Regular pharmacies stock the 50 mg capsules of naltrexone, the dosage prescribed for addictions. But LDN capsules, tablets, liquids, and creams are available only through compounding pharmacies, which create customized dosages of naltrexone for LDN therapy.

With LDN, compounding pharmacies are making what amounts to a different drug entirely: LDN from naltrexone. Not all compounding pharmacies do an equally good job of compounding LDN. Lowdosenaltrexone.org (LDNinfo.org) lists several that have had a great deal of experience compounding LDN from naltrexone, and the list is growing.[37]

LDN is generally taken in dosages of 3 to 4.5 mg, once a day at bedtime. Most people can tolerate this safe dose. According to compounding pharmacist Dr. Skip Lenz, in most cases, sleep disturbances can be easily avoided if the person starts at a lower dosage of 1.5 mg for about one month, titrating[38] up to 3 mg for one month. After that, Dr. Lenz says the patient and the physician should evaluate the situation, and together they can decide whether or not to raise the dose to 4.5 mg. Dr. Lenz feels that for the majority of patients, 3 mg is the optimal dose. The issue of dosage is still up for discussion, however, and a majority of prescribing physicians prefer the 4.5 mg daily dosage of LDN.

So, what about side effects? Patients starting treatment with LDN sometimes report having vivid dreams. That's it. This is not to be confused with side effects for naltrexone prescribed in doses of 50 mg and higher to treat addictions. At these doses, naltrexone can lead to gastrointestinal symptoms and can potentially cause liver damage. The doses are so low with LDN, however, that there is no evidence that it negatively affects the liver.

There is one contraindication for LDN. For patients who are dependent on narcotics, LDN can trigger withdrawal symptoms. Therefore, narcotics must be entirely out of the system before starting LDN. In addition, if a patient is scheduled for surgery where opiates will be given as part of the anesthesia or for pain management after surgery, LDN should be discontinued seven days before surgery. A health professional can determine when it's safe to resume taking LDN, depending on the pain medications that are used and the number of days they are taken.

The Uses of LDN

In *Honest Medicine,* I focused on the successes of patients who used LDN for MS. In this book, I'm focusing on using LDN for MS as well as a wide range of additional autoimmune disorders, including lupus, myasthenia gravis, RA, chronic fatigue syndrome, Hashimoto's thyroiditis, fibromyalgia, and Crohn's disease. I have also included Parkinson's disease because recent data suggest that there is an autoimmune component to Parkinson's. As you will read, Lexie Lindstrom, the Parkinson's patient profiled in this book, reports excellent results with LDN. Thanks to Lexie, many Parkinson's patients—including one doctor in Norway—are now taking and benefiting from LDN.[39]

At this point, we have likely only scratched the surface of what I believe is a significant breakthrough in healthcare, which is why I often call LDN a *cause célèbre*. In *Honest Medicine*, I referred to it as "one of the most important medical discoveries of the twentieth century—if not *the* most important," and Dr. David Gluck calls it "one of the most significant therapeutic discoveries in fifty years." We already see the results with several pioneering doctors and patients being willing to go against standard medical practice and advice to try something new. This "something" also happens to be extremely low-cost, safe, and effective.[40]

Another hero of mine, Burton Berkson, MD, whose work was also profiled in *Honest Medicine*, has consistently reported positive results with LDN among patients. Dr. Berkson uses LDN along with intravenous alpha lipoic acid, an innovative treatment for which he is known worldwide. With this combination, he treats many patients with liver diseases, autoimmune diseases, and some cancers. For a more detailed discussion of Dr. Berkson's work, please read *Honest Medicine* (Chapter 4, pages 65-78).

This is what Dr. Berkson says about Low Dose Naltrexone:

> It is difficult for many to believe that one drug can accomplish so many tasks. But LDN does not treat symptoms as most drugs do. It actually works way "upstream" to modulate the basic mechanisms that result in the disease state.

Why Is It Difficult to Get LDN Prescribed?

Dr. David Gluck has some thoughts about why doctors are so leery about prescribing LDN. As he points out in *Honest Medicine* (Chapter 11, page 193):

> You have to put yourself in the position of the physician. The physician has spent years and years in training. And that training focuses on the scientific method, on making sure that what he is going to use has been shown to work in a scientific way backed up by scientific studies—not from patient stories, which they call "anecdotes." To them, it's got to be in a well-known medical journal; it's got to be peer-reviewed. It has to be tested in large studies—double-blind, placebo-controlled studies. It has to be FDA-approved. But even if it's not FDA-approved for a particular use, doctors do have the right to write an off-label prescription for any dose of something that has been FDA-approved, even if it was approved at a higher dose, like naltrexone was.

The Limited Research on LDN

According to Dr. David Gluck, LDN is overlooked in most medical journals. He says:

> To run the big studies costs millions of dollars...Naltrexone has been off-patent for some years. Pharmaceutical companies run in the other direction when people talk about wanting to run a trial for LDN, because they would put in all that money and find that there are no profits waiting at the other end, since anybody can get the generic naltrexone and break it down into whatever dose they want through a compounding pharmacy at a very low cost.

On to the Revolution!

Clearly, I've only scratched the surface here about LDN's potential to transform the way we approach autoimmune diseases. In the chapters ahead, you'll read stories about women and men from the US and several other countries who faced challenges in getting LDN, but ultimately benefited from taking this drug. These patients speak for themselves, telling their stories in their own words. I continue to be inspired by the many people willing to speak out about their experiences, as a way to help others. I hope you will obtain the information you need to help you decide whether LDN might help you, your family, or friends, along with the inspiration and motivation to successfully seek LDN therapy if you believe it would be potentially helpful to you.

On to the Revolution.

CHAPTER 2

Autoimmune Diseases

*If you listen to the whispers,
you won't have to hear the screams...*
C.S. Lewis

Many thanks to my friend and colleague, Virginia McCullough, for collaborating with me on this chapter.[41]

If you're reading this book, it's a pretty good guess that you or someone close to you has been diagnosed with at least one autoimmune disease or immune system disorder. Because Low Dose Naltrexone (LDN) is a successful treatment for conditions linked to immune system malfunctions, it's important to understand how the immune system works. Ordinarily, the treatments conventional doctors prescribe carry risks, and the relief gained from these treatments is often accompanied by side effects ranging from mildly unpleasant to severe—and even unbearable. In some cases, these drugs carry "side effects" as severe as the deadly brain infection, progressive multifocal leukoencephalopathy (PML) and cancers, such as lymphomas.

But, as you already know from previous chapters, LDN works differently—and gently—to successfully treat many autoimmune and other conditions.

First, it's important to note that a healthy immune system is crucial to our health; it is what keeps our bodies working correctly.

When our immune system fails to work properly, we're more likely to become ill. This complex system has been likened to sentry guards or a border patrol—or, in modern terms, to an antivirus program that protects our computers. No matter what terms and analogies we use to define it, the immune system's primary job is to identify and protect us from invaders that threaten us—invaders such as bacteria, viruses, parasites, chemicals, and mold. When it works correctly, this extraordinarily complex system spots invaders and puts seek-and-destroy actions into motion. If this isn't possible, it constructs barriers to protect vulnerable organs and tissues.

Put simply, the immune system's job is to distinguish between "us" and "them," or "self" and "not self." When it's working well, the immune system sees "self" and calls it "safe." In contrast, "not self" signals "unsafe."

In order to protect the body, your immune system must have a way to identify potential dangers. Fortunately, substances such as bacteria, viruses, pet dander, chemicals, and parasites all have markers, called antigens, that signal their presence. These antigens are what your immune system responds to as "not self" and therefore, "not safe."

Clearly, this is an over-simplification. Suffice it to say the immune system is complicated and is working every nanosecond we're alive. It's always adjusting, adapting, and producing antibodies in reaction to the antigens that threaten it. The immune system goes into high gear when we face a threat such as chemical exposure, bacterial invasion, or an allergen like pollen or a cat's dander. When the threat subsides, the immune system throttles back.

The immune system accomplishes its job through various types of lymphoid organs, such as the spleen and lymph nodes, along with a variety of specialized cells our bodies produce to perform unique functions. All these cells are powerful and interdependent. Examples include macrophages, which act as front-line defenders against bacteria, viruses, and other invaders; and basophils, which are activated in acute immune system response to an allergen.

Some immune system cells take on a search-and-destroy mission and never allow the invader access to tissues and organs in the first place. For instance, the rhinovirus—the cause of the common cold—produces symptoms that make us miserable for a few days, but most often we recover quickly and without complications. Or, we might successfully fight off a cold, but for reasons we don't fully understand, our spouse, children, or next-door neighbor might not be so lucky. In any case, the common cold usually doesn't last long. Not so with other conditions, such as the autoimmune diseases discussed in this book.

When the body detects an invader, various types of immune system cells perceive a threat. To combat that threat, they increase in number and create protective barriers that produce inflammation. The redness and swelling that forms around a skin wound, for example, is the body's inflammatory response to an injury. When it's working well and is not overwhelmed, the immune system helps us stay well and recover from illnesses when they occur.

Autoimmune Disease, an Immune System Disorder

The immune system can develop disorders, such as the autoimmune conditions featured in this book, which interfere with its ability to function as it should *for long periods of time*. According to the American Autoimmune Related Diseases Association (AARDA), the first association to address these conditions as a group, autoimmune conditions affect at least 50 million Americans. No one has yet pinpointed the exact reasons why the body's defense mechanisms are marshaled to respond to cells within the body as if they were dangerous, foreign invaders. With an autoimmune disease, it's as if the controls the body normally uses to distinguish "self" and "not self" are interrupted and lose their ability to function normally.

Some autoimmune disorders are organ-specific. For example, both Hashimoto's thyroiditis and Graves' disease target the thyroid gland; Addison's disease targets the adrenal glands; and autoimmune hepatitis targets the liver. On the other hand, many other autoimmune disorders are systemic, meaning that the autoimmune activity is spread throughout the body. Lupus and rheumatoid arthritis (RA) are two examples of systemic diseases. They affect various tissues throughout the body and produce a variety of symptoms. It is not surprising, then, that many patients have difficulty getting a correct diagnosis because of the array of symptoms these diseases can produce.

Many autoimmune diseases also have some symptoms in common. On March 1, 2016, Autoimmunemom.com, a popular website and blog created by Katie Cleary, featured a guest post by Gretchen Heber, titled "12 Super Symptoms of Autoimmune Disease."[42] Heber lists symptoms that are common to several autoimmune diseases, including inflammation, persistent low-grade fever, extreme fatigue, swollen glands, and tingling. This posting reinforces the fact that autoimmune diseases can be extremely difficult to diagnosis.

In addition—and this is a huge problem—no medical specialty exists that is devoted to the study of autoimmune diseases, so no one group of doctors specializes in their treatments. A patient would see an endocrinologist for autoimmune thyroid conditions, a rheumatologist for rheumatoid arthritis, a gastroenterologist for Crohn's, an allergist for asthma, a neurologist for multiple sclerosis (MS) and Parkinson's, and other specialists for other conditions.

Looking at the Numbers

While it's almost impossible to cite exact numbers of people who have been diagnosed with any one of the many autoimmune diseases, most likely AARDA's estimate of 50 million Americans is correct. However, since more diseases are being classified as autoimmune all the time, by the time you are reading this book, this estimate will undoubtedly be outdated.[43]

Worldwide, the same alarming trends are becoming increasingly apparent. While it's true that autoimmune disorders develop among all populations, they appear to occur in greater numbers in industrialized, Western countries. And while no one can provide absolute numbers, it's safe to say that autoimmune diseases negatively affect the lives of many millions of people throughout the world.

A Relatively New Science

What we know about autoimmune diseases seems to come in waves as patients, research institutions and doctors from various specialties share information. However, research into autoimmune diseases continues to run into obstacles that prevent them from being understood and viewed as connected to a group of causes or mechanisms.

The first scientist to address autoimmune diseases was Noel Rose, MD, who identified the phenomenon of autoimmunity in the 1950s,[44] but many of the diseases we now know as autoimmune have been with us far longer. We just didn't understand them or realize that the immune system was the root of their cause. The concept of autoimmunity wasn't fully accepted until the 1960s and '70s, and even now, most scientists agree that these diseases aren't well understood, individually or as a group.

Dr. Rose did his breakthrough work during a time when the study of immunity was not a particularly popular research area. Author Donna Jackson Nakazawa, in her book *The Autoimmune Epidemic*,[45] explains that in the early 1900s, Paul Ehrlich, PhD, a German immunologist, researcher, and Nobel laureate, declared it impossible for the immune system to attack the body's healthy tissues—and that, he said, was that. Dr. Ehrlich's belief spread throughout the scientific community and stood unchallenged for half a century. However, Dr. Rose's research, conducted at the State University of New York at Buffalo, reversed these entrenched beliefs.

By 1957, Dr. Rose's experiments revealed that in Hashimoto's thyroiditis, the immune system attacked the cells of the thyroid gland. Despite this, it wasn't until the late 1960s that the concept of autoimmune disorders gained wide acceptance in the medical community. Dr. Rose himself continued his life's work, eventually becoming the Director of the Center for Autoimmune Research at the Johns Hopkins' School of Medicine and at Hopkins' Bloomberg School of Public Health, where he remains today. Dr. Rose is also a professor of molecular microbiology and immunology at Johns Hopkins, as well as a professor of pathology at the university's School of Medicine.[46]

Many obstacles remain. From the point of view of patients, the diagnostic process is not only problematic; it can be nightmarish. Worse, standard drug treatments bring inconsistent and unpredictable results in controlling symptoms, and these drugs tend to be expensive. To quote from *The Cost Burden of Autoimmune Disease: The Latest Front in the War on Healthcare Spending*,[47] a joint publication of the National Coalition of Autoimmune Patient Groups and AARDA: "In 2001, National Institutes of Allergy and Infectious Diseases (NIAID) Director Dr. Anthony Fauci estimated that annual autoimmune disease treatment costs were greater than $100 billion." And that estimate, the publication suggests, is low.

Looking at costs on a more personal level, the conventional treatment of autoimmune disorders is such an expensive undertaking that it's often out of reach for the uninsured. In many cases, even those with adequate coverage often find that their insurance covers doctors' visits and prescription drugs, but doesn't cover potentially helpful alternative treatments such as acupuncture, nutritional supplements, or massage therapy. In other words, patients are steered toward the more conventional—and often more expensive and toxic—treatments, while a lesser-known or less conventional treatment such as LDN is often not mentioned by conventional doctors and won't be covered by insurance.

This disparity in coverage confuses many people, but the reason for it goes back to the way drugs are approved. The pharmaceuticals prescribed by doctors for autoimmune conditions are often toxic and expensive, sometimes costing as much as $60,000 per patient per year—or even more. Still, they have been approved by the FDA based on findings in large clinical trials. That sounds reasonable, but there's a catch. More often than not, these trials have been paid for by pharmaceutical companies that manufacture and sell the drugs they are testing—a definite conflict of interest. (You can find an excellent discussion of this problem in Dr. David Gluck's chapter in *Honest Medicine*.)

This explains why most insurance policies will not cover LDN, which costs—depending on the compounding pharmacy that makes it—*around a dollar a day, or even less*, and has virtually no side effects.

Based on the current conventional medical "wisdom," pharmaceutical medications for autoimmune conditions are developed with the goal of suppressing the immune system, so it will stop attacking itself. Pharmaceutical drugs currently used to treat these diseases do just that. However, because these drugs successfully suppress the immune system, they leave the body susceptible to developing other extremely serious conditions, including certain cancers.

Dr. Bihari saw things differently. In *Honest Medicine*, Mary Boyle Bradley describes how Dr. Bihari's approach to autoimmune diseases flew in the face of the commonly held medical wisdom. He reasoned that the immune systems of people with these conditions needed *strengthening*, rather than suppressing. According to Dr. Bihari, LDN "modulates" or "orchestrates" the immune system, causing it to function correctly. [Author's Note: For an excellent explanation of how LDN works, see Dr. David Gluck's chapter in *Honest Medicine*—Chapter 11—as well as a fascinating video interview with Dr. Bihari that was first posted on my website, HonestMedicine.com.[48] The transcription was later published, with my permission, in *Alternative Therapies Magazine*.[49]]

In any case, the fact that the action of this inexpensive, off-label drug flies in the face of conventional medical "wisdom" is one of the reasons conventional doctors find LDN so challenging to understand, and therefore to accept and prescribe.

In the chapters ahead, patients tell about the terrible side effects they experienced with the conventional pharmaceuticals prescribed for their autoimmune disorders—side effects and complications drug companies often admit to in their television and print ads. For example, many of the warnings at the end of TV ads for drugs like Humira—used to treat the symptoms of conditions such as rheumatoid arthritis (RA), Crohn's disease, and plaque psoriasis—are dire. The same is true for Enbrel, used to treat several forms of arthritis; and Lyrica, used for fibromyalgia and diabetic nerve pain. Orencia, another drug used for RA, also warns of severe side effects. We could make our way through a long list of medications, risks, and common side effects. [Author's Note: The approved uses for these drugs are always expanding as the drug companies that manufacture them conduct more clinical trials on their drugs' uses for additional autoimmune diseases.]

An example: One AbbVie TV ad states that Humira helps to relieve rheumatoid arthritis pain and protect joints "from further damage." However, at the end of the commercial comes the warning that the drug "can lower your ability to fight infections, including tuberculosis. Serious, sometimes fatal infections and cancers, including lymphoma, have happened, as have blood, liver, and nervous system problems, serious allergic reactions, and new or worsening heart failure."[50] Some television commercials and print ads even list "death" as a possible side effect.

Wow! Some "side effects!"

Autoimmune Diseases on the Rise

Since the 1960s, one disease after another has made its way into discussions of autoimmune diseases, which now include well over 100 distinct conditions. The medical community eventually recognized some diseases, such as MS, RA, and lupus as autoimmune disorders, and today, the general public increasingly recognizes them as a group of related diseases.

Some of these autoimmune conditions—e.g., MS and lupus—are also neurological conditions, and hence, treated by a neurologist. On the other hand, Hashimoto's thyroiditis and Graves' disease are treated by endocrinologists; rheumatoid arthritis by rheumatologists; and Crohn's disease by gastroenterologists. So, even when people have heard of these diseases, they don't necessarily link them or see them as related. At first glance, Hashimoto's thyroiditis and Crohn's disease appear to have little in common, but that just isn't true. Although most of us have heard of MS, psoriasis, chronic fatigue syndrome (CFS), and RA, fewer of us are familiar with polymyalgia rheumatica or a more recently identified autoimmune disease called antiphospholipid antibody syndrome (APS). Today, we can identify a virtual alphabet soup of dozens of these autoimmune conditions.

As you will see, this book features stories about a handful of mostly well-known autoimmune diseases that were treated successfully with LDN. Just because an autoimmune disease isn't mentioned doesn't mean it's insignificant, or that it won't respond to LDN. To explore this further, please see Linda Elsegood's list of 200+ conditions—many of which are autoimmune—that might be helped by LDN.[51]

The Complexity of Autoimmune Diseases

As mentioned earlier, despite their number and the vast array of reported symptoms, autoimmune diseases have some commonalities when we look at them closely, including some shared symptoms or even large symptom clusters. Unfortunately—to make matters even more confusing—not all the conditions have the same symptoms. If that were the case, it might be easier to reach a correct diagnosis quickly and efficiently. However, precisely because so many symptoms are involved, diagnosis and treatment can be complex; so complex, in fact, that seeking professional help and coping with symptoms while waiting for correct answers—sometimes for years—can become a fulltime job.

Since the 100+ known autoimmune diseases are not treated by a specialist in autoimmune diseases, they generally are diagnosed and treated through a complicated referral process. So, if the majority of your symptoms involve joint pain and intractable fatigue, your primary care physician will likely refer you to a rheumatologist. If you are experiencing digestive symptoms, you probably will be referred to a gastroenterologist. If you have numbness and tingling in your hands and feet and MS is suspected, you'll probably be sent to a neurologist. But again, your doctor's referral may not be to the correct specialist.

Mary Shomon, bestselling author of several books on thyroid disease as well as *Living Well with Autoimmune Disease*,[52] cites figures collected by the AARDA that show the difficulties people encounter when they try to discover the root cause of their debilitating symptoms. For example, she reports that in 1996, a typical patient with an autoimmune disorder saw six doctors over a period of six years before receiving a correct diagnosis and subsequent treatment. By 2001, that number dropped to an average of five doctors in five years. Averages, however, don't tell the entire story. Some patients will see 10 doctors in five years or five doctors in three years. No matter how long people search for answers, as their symptoms progress, their daily lives become more difficult.

AARDA's statistics don't take into account the endless search for answers from *other* healthcare professionals such as chiropractors, massage therapists, naturopaths, acupuncturists, and nutritionists, not to mention psychotherapists, hypnotherapists, or yoga or meditation practitioners.

Sadly, some people end up abandoning their quest for help. Financially and/or emotionally, they just can't afford visits to yet one more specialist, or they are completely worn out and discouraged by their failure to find answers. Sometimes they withdraw and attempt to cope on their own without medical help. Their goal becomes learning to *coexist* with their symptoms, ultimately finding ways to work around them.

For better or worse, autoimmune diseases are often invisible with no outward symptoms, so patients might be coping in silence while showing no visible signs of illness. Columnist Arlene Grau, who has fibromyalgia herself, expressed this beautifully in her column titled "Miss Understood: Fibromyalgia Ignorance Hurts."[53] She wrote: "When I first read about the symptoms of fibromyalgia, I was skeptical. How could my body tell me I'm in extreme pain when it seemed like nothing was wrong with me? Why did I look normal on the outside but feel like I was on fire?"

The Brush-Off

Since *Honest Medicine* was published in 2011, I have been a guest on over two hundred radio and Internet talk shows—many of them call-in shows. One after another, listeners have told me about what boils down to "the brush-off." This is the easy dismissal by doctors of symptoms that are difficult to assess and diagnose. Because autoimmune disorders often have overlapping symptoms and so many combinations exist, it's easy to dismiss a patient's symptoms as somehow temporary, even "normal." For example, people have told me about doctors who said:

- "You just had a baby; give it time. All new mothers are tired—even depressed."
- "Your hands are numb, and you get headaches? Stay away from the computer for a few days."
- "Well, of course you're anxious and depressed. You just lost your job (or spouse, home, pet, parent, sibling). We'll try antidepressants—short term—to help you through this bad time."
- "Fatigue, insomnia, muscle aches. Hmm…sounds like premenstrual syndrome (or menopause)."
- "Since we can't find any physical cause, your symptoms are probably stress-related. We have counselors on staff. We'll set up an intake appointment."

As in the above examples, patients' symptoms are often explained away by doctors as the result of hormones or life stress. But that doesn't make the symptoms less problematic. All too often, the easier explanations lead to pigeonholing symptoms so as to fit into preconceived diagnostic labels. Then, when the patients don't get better with the standard treatments for their incorrectly diagnosed conditions, they get the brush-off.

There is another factor that contributes to the brush-off. Since women make up 75 to 80 percent of patients with autoimmune diseases, we can't ignore the tendency to minimize or even dismiss women's symptoms as psychological—or even imagined. Several of the above examples speak to this prejudice. But men's complaints, too, are often brushed off as being "psychological" or "in your head." A full 50 percent of women and men say that during their years-long search for help they were often told that nothing was wrong with them. According to the AARDA, 45 percent of patients with autoimmune diseases say they've been labeled as hypochondriacs.[54] No wonder so many people coping with autoimmune diseases report feeling marginalized and even stigmatized by their illness!

The brush-off by doctors is one thing. But just as troubling is the fact that many people with autoimmune diseases have told me they suffer terribly when even their families and friends lose patience. And this is probably made worse when the disease itself—for instance, fibromyalgia or chronic fatigue syndrome—is often seen by doctors as "suspect," or "not a real disease," and those who suffer from these conditions are viewed suspiciously as hypochondriacs. Several of the people profiled in this book have told me their family members didn't even believe they were ill—because, after all, they were going to the "best doctors," and those doctors were treating them with the "best drugs" and even then, the patients weren't improving! When they finally found LDN—and improved—many family members were genuinely surprised.

Most of the patients profiled in this book suffered symptoms for several years and visited one doctor after another before being correctly diagnosed. For example, it took many years before Darlene Nichols was diagnosed with lupus and then developed myasthenia gravis. It was several more years before she found LDN, which changed her life by completely reversing both conditions. The same is true for Lexie Lindstrom (Parkinson's disease), as well as for Renée Foster (fibromyalgia), Maureen Mirand (RA), John O'Connell (Hashimoto's), Maija Haavisto (chronic fatigue syndrome), and others profiled in this book.

The reasons for the higher prevalence of autoimmune disorders among women are not yet clear. Collectively, however, these diseases affect women's lives more than many of the conditions that have become known as significant concerns for women, such as breast cancer and heart disease. To put this in perspective, in the US, over two million women live with breast cancer, and over seven million live with heart disease, but almost 10 million women have one of the top seven autoimmune diseases. Until I began looking at autoimmune diseases, I didn't realize that taken together they form the eighth leading cause of death for women in the US.

Among both men and women, autoimmune diseases are the second leading cause of chronic illness and the third most common reason cited for filing for Social Security Disability. Illness is costly, and not just in economic terms. Unlike some of the degenerative illnesses such as cancer, heart disease, and osteoarthritis—whose incidence rises with age—many autoimmune diseases strike younger people in what is supposed to be the prime of their lives. Although the numbers are not precise, about one in nine women of child-bearing age will deal with at least one autoimmune disease, and it is not uncommon for people to suffer from more than one.

I've heard so many heartbreaking accounts of young women and men whose careers were severely compromised or cut short because of MS, Hashimoto's disease, Parkinson's, lupus, or other conditions profiled in this book. And it goes without saying that these diseases adversely affect family life. Autoimmune diseases almost always mean some degree of accommodation and adjustment, and often major life changes. Economic costs aside, the human toll is devastating, and it's getting worse.

Rising Rates—the U.S. is Not Alone

The incidence of autoimmune diseases is definitely on the rise in Western countries. Because these illnesses haven't been addressed by one medical specialty, the numbers have sometimes been scattered and unconnected. Consequently, doctors and patients alike miss the bigger picture. However, no matter how we measure it, we know for sure that autoimmune diseases are becoming more common in Western countries.

The Mayo Clinic reports that the incidence of lupus has tripled over the last 40 years, and while, again, the incidence is higher in women than in men, African American women are at even higher risk of developing it. I could cite statistics from every Northern European country that show stark increases in rates of MS over the last 40 to 50 years, generally an annual increase of three percent.

Alone in a Crowd

Western societies, perhaps especially the United States, tend to promote the happiness to be found in living fully, working hard, and playing hard. We say we value health, productivity, family life, and all that goes into the aggressive pursuit of achievement and happiness. In this atmosphere, we run the risk of looking at illness as a weakness or failure.

We spend millions of dollars annually immunizing ourselves against threatening invaders like polio, diphtheria, mumps, measles, and many other infectious diseases that historically appeared as epidemics, rather than in scattered, isolated cases. While attention was focused on developing vaccines to prevent epidemics, autoimmune diseases have been steadily rising, causing untold personal and economic hardship. While the increase in autoimmune diseases doesn't match the precise medical definition of an epidemic, we're certainly in the midst of an emergency, even if we haven't labeled it as such.

Autoimmune diseases can be devastating, and not only because of delayed diagnosis and treatment. Although autoimmune disorders are often invisible, their symptoms can affect every aspect of daily life. I've spoken with many people whose day-to-day lives were marked by debilitating pain, crushing fatigue, digestive distress, mental fogginess, inability to focus, insomnia, and depression. And the list goes on. Some of their symptoms resulted from the prescribed treatments, which cause difficult-to-handle side effects and also come with risks of their own. Furthermore, the conditions the drugs are meant to treat often don't substantially improve; in fact, sometimes they get worse with the drugs.

In spite of the challenges they face, the women and men I've met through my website (HonestMedicine.com), Facebook, email, radio shows, and teleseminars and coaching sessions are also among the most courageous people I've ever known. It can be lonely to have an illness that few understand and that often produces symptoms that are written off as imaginary, or exaggerated, or stress-related. Yet, the people whose stories appear in this book have persevered. They kept looking for answers and eventually found them, but rarely from their doctors. Most often, they discovered LDN on their own through online research and support groups. It's no wonder that several of the contributors to *Honest Medicine* and this book proclaimed: "Thank goodness for the Internet!"

LDN reduces autoimmune symptoms and can stop the progression of diseases—a major breakthrough and advance in medicine.

This advance is even more exciting because patients themselves are speaking up about the benefits of LDN. As more people learn about the effectiveness and safety of LDN—plus its low cost and the absence of side effects—word will spread more quickly, and many more patients will be helped.

SECTION II:

THE LDN HEROES

CHAPTER 3

Fritz Bell (GoodShape.net)

I first learned about Fritz Bell (aka "GoodShape") from Mary Boyle Bradley, who shared her husband Noel's experience with LDN in Honest Medicine. *Mary first learned about LDN in 2002 from GoodShape.net, a website created and run by Fritz. The website also had a message board for people eager to learn about alternative multiple sclerosis treatments and to share their experiences. (The website was active from 2000 to 2015.)*

Mary began communicating with others on the board, as well as with Fritz, who told her that, ever since his wife Polly began taking LDN for her MS in 2000, she experienced almost immediate improvement and never had another exacerbation. Mary decided to convince Noel to try it. So, it was because of Fritz that Noel started taking LDN, and was helped for many years.

From 2011 to 2012, Mary had a BlogTalkRadio program devoted entirely to LDN. She interviewed many of the pioneers, including Drs. David Gluck and Ian Zagon. She also interviewed Fritz, as well as many other LDN patient advocates, including SammyJo Wilkinson, Destiny Marquez, and me.

I met Fritz at an LDN conference in Chicago in 2013, and we became friends. I learned the dramatic story of how LDN helped Polly, and how their experience turned Fritz into a tireless and passionate advocate for LDN. He has convinced many people to try it and has, in fact, helped just as many to make their own LDN.

As you will see from his story, Fritz was one of the early LDN pioneers. I am honored that he has agreed to tell his story for our book. His chapter is taken in part, with Mary's permission, from her BlogTalkRadio interview with Fritz.

Here is Fritz's story in his own words.

My late wife Polly was originally diagnosed with MS in 1986. From then, until we found LDN in 2000, her condition declined. By 1995, she needed a wheelchair. We experienced what many people have gone through—the panic that nothing is working.

Out of desperation, we got in line early for Betaseron, the CRAB drug that came on the market in 1996. But in our case, as in many others, the drug was a disaster. Polly went backward as soon as she got on Betaseron. It took us about two or three months to realize this, but once we figured it out, I started searching and looking for other options. [Author's Note: CRAB drugs are four "disease-modifying drugs," often prescribed as the first line of treatment for MS patients. CRAB stands for Copaxone, Rebif, Avonex, and Betaseron.]

In September 1999, people on the message board found a transdermal histamine treatment, which afforded Polly and a few other people on the board some measure of improved energy. But Polly and others didn't experience true improvement until LDN.

Many of the people who participated in my message board had been kicked off regular medical message boards for spouting alternative medicine ideas, which weren't popular in those days. Somehow or other, quite a bunch—maybe a dozen people, who had some really good alternative medicine ideas—ended up on the GoodShape board.

At that time, message board members used made-up names—for instance, there were Norma AK from Alaska, Marilyn from Vancouver, Marlene from Washington, and Jeannie Z from Florida. These people ended up helping me to oversee the board.

I don't know who heard about LDN first, but I do remember that one of us discovered an article from the winter of 1999 that had been published in the Brewer Science Library Newsletter out of Wisconsin. It was an un-authored article, but we soon discovered that it was written by a woman named Christina L. White—a brilliant alternative medicine researcher and writer.

In the article, Christina White wrote that she had interviewed a friend of Dr. Bihari's daughter, to whom he had given Low Dose Naltrexone a dozen years before for multiple sclerosis. The story goes that this young woman reportedly took LDN for her MS for 10 years, then stopped taking it when she went out of state, and her supply ran out. She ended up getting an exacerbation about three or four weeks later that landed her in the hospital. According to the article, she went back on LDN and was doing well again. A very impressive story about the power of LDN!

Christina L. White's article ended with something like, "It's too bad things like this take 10 or 15 years to develop and test. But wouldn't it be nice if somebody out there would test it themselves? And if you do, please write me a letter and tell me how it worked for you."

A number of us on that message board were excited about doing just that; we took up the challenge, and by early March 2000, a dozen or so of us were taking LDN. And we didn't begin at 1 mg. We jumped right in at 4.5 mg! We didn't know any better. Within a month, all of the people who took LDN were reporting a level of success and were planning to continue taking it. Several of us are taking it to this day.

Polly started taking LDN at the beginning of March 2000 and had an excellent response to it. Before LDN, she had pretty much been in bed for all but an hour or two a day and was only getting up in her wheelchair for dinner. But within a couple of days, she was sleeping better and waking up better. The first couple of nights at 4.5 mg were a little rough, but within a matter of days, things were going more smoothly. Our life picked up. We took two cruises and went back to going shopping and all kinds of things we hadn't been able to do for some time. Polly returned to a level of activity she hadn't experienced for at least five years.

Unfortunately, she died from heart failure at age 65, four years after starting LDN. Heart conditions were in her family's history, but she lived 10 years longer than others in her immediate family. When she died, Polly's MS had been stable for four years, and we were planning our third recovery cruise.

I credit her dramatically improved functionality and quality of life to LDN. Polly's and my experience with LDN, as well as the experiences of many of the people on our message board, turned me into a patient advocate—dedicated to helping others to get LDN.

In the early years I gave away a lot of 50 mg Revia naltrexone tablets along with amber bottles, droppers and instructions to create homemade liquid LDN. Today, I give out Naltrexone from two American manufacturers. But now that I am getting older, I have slowed the fight.

But, over the years, I have been able to help many people by providing them with LDN. Here are several of my recollections.

In 2005, I was a guest speaker at the inaugural "Low Dose Naltrexone Annual Conference" in New York City. There, I spoke about the first major LDN-facilitated cancer recovery that I witnessed. There were to be many others after that.

In 2004, a friend called me at our Florida home and said that her 88-year-old father was dying of terminal prostate cancer; he had been in a coma and sent home from the hospital with hospice care. She wondered if it was too late to try "that medicine you always talk about" on her father. With nothing to lose, I provided her with a bottle of liquid LDN and told her to put a few drops into his permanently open mouth every evening. I left town the next day to spend the summer up north.

When I returned to Florida in December, this woman called to ask me to come to dinner the following Friday. I accepted and apologized for not having checked in with her for news of her father. She said not to worry, and that she would tell me about him at dinner. Shortly after I arrived, to my utter shock and delight, her father and mother walked in the door, having just returned from a cruise. After three weeks in a coma and on intravenous feeding, a few drops of LDN over four evenings caused him to wake up and announce that he wanted milk!

I understand that his doctors all dismissed his LDN treatment as having been of no value. He lived another four years. To my knowledge, his prostate cancer never returned.

A few years later this same friend convinced her brother to take LDN two weeks before scheduled surgery to remove intestines that had been damaged by Crohn's disease. But when he entered the hospital for his pre-op examinations, his physicians sent him home: They could not find the damaged area they planned to remove.

A woman from the GoodShape message board who had received medicine from me wrote me a long email describing a June visit the previous year she had had with her sister and her 15-year-old nephew. They had been to see the oncologist who was treating the young man's glioblastoma, a fast-growing and often fatal brain tumor.

During the visit, the family was advised that the oncologist had exhausted all options for the 15-year-old and informed his mother that it was unlikely that he would make it to the end of the year. At that time, the woman offered her sister—the patient's mother—naltrexone tablets and the preparation materials I had given her. He began taking LDN shortly after that devastating doctor's visit.

The following March, the young man returned to the oncologist's office with his mother and aunt. The doctor reviewed the recent CT scans of his brain. Upon first look, he saw no signs of the glioblastoma. According to the email the boy's aunt sent me, the physician left the examining room and brought back three other oncologists who observed the boy, commented on the scans, and had a discussion in the hall. The young man's oncologist returned and announced that the doctors had agreed that they would write up this boy's incredible remission in their hospital newsletter as the first such miracle that had taken place that year in the hospital's cancer unit.

The young man's miraculous remission from a glioblastoma was chronicled a couple of months later. But, of course, there was no mention of his elective LDN treatment. That story made me cry—with happiness.

Another family friend had a 45-year-old son with multiple myeloma, an incurable blood cancer. The family spent hundreds of thousands of dollars on chemotherapy treatments and all kinds of other treatments to arrest this disease—all to no avail. Ultimately, he was bedridden at his elderly parents' home. Many visitors came to say their goodbyes. I gave his sister the usual amber bottle containing liquid LDN and suggested that she give him a few drops every night.

The story I got a couple of weeks later was simply amazing.

After four days on the LDN treatment, this man miraculously got out of bed. He dressed himself and came downstairs for breakfast to meet with some of his farewell visitors. His mother was so amazed by his apparent recovery that she called his oncologist to get him back on chemotherapy. Neither the mother nor her son's physician believed that the LDN treatment was of any importance. He returned to chemotherapy and unfortunately, did not survive. That story made me cry because it was so incredibly sad.

After years of vacationing in Michigan, I became acquainted with a cleaning woman in her sixties who had some drinking and smoking habits. When I saw her one June, she told me that both she and her husband had undergone treatment for lung cancer. She also told me that her 40-year-old son had committed suicide during that summer and that she had decided against further cancer treatments. She felt that she could no longer go on. I asked her if she would do me one big favor, and I gave her a six-month supply of naltrexone tablets to make her own LDN, along with directions on how to prepare and take it. She promised me she would take it and keep me informed.

In December she called, asking for more naltrexone and told me she had not felt this good in over two years. She was unloading truckloads of firewood and baking Christmas cookies for the first time in years. Her husband, who had not taken LDN, died from lung cancer the following summer. She was still doing well eight years later and moved to another state. I eventually lost touch with her but was glad to have helped her have a second chance at life.

My college roommate and good friend was diagnosed with primary lateral sclerosis, a disease similar to the dreaded ALS, twelve years ago. He became a permanent LDN user and is now one of my healthiest friends! He still walks with a limp but plays golf three times a week and has "shot his age" several times.

I know two elderly men who were both diagnosed with stage four prostate cancer and have been taking LDN for ten years. They do not know each other, but I have followed their progress and am happy to report that both are doing very well, with an excellent quality of life. One lives down the street from me, and the other lives on the west coast of Florida. Both men retired because their doctors predicted that they only had months to live. One of these men was a promising new president of a state university, but his career was cut short after this serious diagnosis. Every time I get reports from these men, I receive the same update: Their oncologists are still telling them that they have stage four prostate cancer and should prepare for the end.

I began my own LDN treatment in March of 2000, at the same time I started Polly on it. I wanted to test it for myself in hopes of preventing future disease. I believe LDN saved me from getting prostate cancer. Before I started taking LDN, my PSA level was high. After LDN, it's been low. As a matter of fact, today, it's lower than it was seventeen years ago. And LDN may have saved me from getting some other minor illnesses. I am sure it has cured my lifetime problem of hypoglycemia. After having avoided sugar my entire life, now I can have a stack of pancakes and syrup! I am making up for some pleasures I missed in my youth and still maintaining my LDN regimen, seventeen years later.

My most recent LDN success story involves my son Christopher's partner Kristen, who was diagnosed with both neuromyelitis optica (or Devic's disease) and myasthenia gravis. She couldn't see anything out of her left eye, and she couldn't see color out of her right eye. After six months of taking LDN, her vision in both eyes improved substantially, and now, she sees normally in each eye. Unfortunately, before finding LDN, she ran up huge hospital bills, because of doctor-prescribed plasmapheresis treatments that didn't help her achieve the remission that LDN gave her.

The good news about LDN keeps spreading through the Internet and the medical world, thanks to organizations like LDN Research Trust and endless Internet postings by dozens of intelligent, caring people like Linda Elsegood, Julia Schopick, Brian Haviland, and Dudley Delany. Thanks to the growing number of doctors like Bob Lawrence, Burt Berkson, Jill Smith, and many others, the work of Dr. Bihari and Dr. David Gluck continues, and an ever-higher level of respect is being generated for this truly remarkable, lifesaving medication. I am genuinely pleased to watch the slow but growing recognition that LDN is securing.

Just recently, I had an opportunity to watch the streaming videos of the LDN conference put on in Portland, Oregon, by Linda

Elsegood and the LDN Research Trust. I was encouraged to watch the presentations by over 30 doctors who are now using LDN successfully in their practices. Add to this the fact that there have been several books about LDN—also a good sign—books like Julia Schopick's *Honest Medicine*, Linda Elsegood's *The LDN Book*, SammyJo Wilkinson's and Elaine Moore's *The Promise of LDN Therapy* and, of course, Mary Boyle Bradley's *Up the Creek with a Paddle*. And now, I am happy to be a part of this new book about LDN.

All of these are wonderful signs that LDN is becoming widely accepted. I believe the possibilities of what LDN can do for people with autoimmune diseases and cancers are endless, and I am happy to have played a part.

It's been almost 20 years since Fritz Bell first learned about LDN, and 18 years since his late wife Polly started using it. Since then, he has helped scores of people get and be helped by this treatment. Fritz has played a huge part in spreading the word about LDN, which is why I call him an LDN Hero.

CHAPTER 4

Christina White (Brewer Science Library), the First Journalist to Write About LDN

I first learned of Christina White from Fritz Bell (GoodShape.net), one of the early LDN pioneers, and a contributor to this book. In Fritz's chapter, he tells how his first introduction to LDN was from reading an article by Christina in the Brewer Science Library newsletter: http://www.mwt.net/~drbrewer/Naltrexone_1.htm.

In her foreword to this book, while she does not refer to Christina by name, Jackie Bihari writes that the Brewer Science Library newsletter was one of the first publications to support Dr. Bihari's work with LDN.

I was surprised to learn that Christina had not been interviewed before this for any of the books about LDN, so I am delighted that she has agreed to be part of this book.

As you will see, the story of her interest in LDN and her relationship with Dr. Bihari is fascinating.

Christina shares her story here.

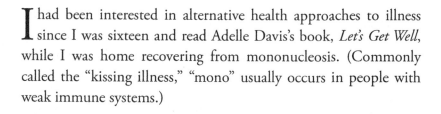

I had been interested in alternative health approaches to illness since I was sixteen and read Adelle Davis's book, *Let's Get Well*, while I was home recovering from mononucleosis. (Commonly called the "kissing illness," "mono" usually occurs in people with weak immune systems.)

I was so impressed with Ms. Davis's results treating people with nutrition and supplements that, in college, I considered becoming a nutritionist. But my guidance counselor talked me into becoming a social studies teacher for junior high and high school instead. When I did my student teaching in a poverty-stricken area of a major city, I was profoundly affected by the poor nutrition many of my students had, which I believed contributed to their academic inadequacies and compromised their future success.

I have always had a deep love of learning and have been an avid reader since childhood. Passing on valuable and often life-saving information through my teaching and writing has been one of the goals and joys of my life.

In the '60s, I frequented a large health food store in the Chicago area where I first learned of Hans A. Nieper, MD, a German physician who treated many Americans—including famous people such as Ronald Reagan—for cancer, heart disease, and multiple sclerosis (MS). Little did I know at the time that this knowledge would eventually lead me to a future job.

Years of life later, my husband and I left Chicago and moved to rural Wisconsin where we live on 43 acres. There I frequented the large public library. I was astonished to discover that on the second floor was a specialty library, the Brewer Science Library, which housed the archives of Dr. Hans Nieper.

Many years later, in 1996, after running some government-funded programs for disadvantaged, low-income youth, adults and seniors, I started working at this specialty library. I was truly delighted to be back in the alternative health field and immediately began digging into research on multiple sclerosis. You see, Dr. Nieper's treatment of MS was the primary interest of the hundreds of people who called us from all over the world to purchase our informational packet about his therapies. They also asked how to contact him.

Dr. Nieper's treatment of MS involved two to three weekly injections or intravenous infusions of Ca-EAP (calcium EAP) for five to seven years, along with some oral supplements designed to go with his protocol.

(Note: There is some confusion as to whether the correct term is calcium EAP or calcium AEP—also Ca-EAP or ca-AEP. Please read the following link for an explanation. https://www.mscenter.org/education/patient-resources/complementary-care/87-in-dietary-supplements/449-calcium-eap)

Most MS patients opted to travel to Germany for a ten-day stay where they obtained daily injections directly from Dr. Nieper. Some patients, who found it difficult to travel to Germany, preferred to have an American physician initiate the therapy, although—because it wasn't an FDA-approved, standard-of-care treatment—it was difficult to find doctors here willing to do this.

Many people benefited immensely from the Nieper therapy for MS, although there was certainly a group that did not. His insistence on the need to continue the therapy for five to seven years proved to be too difficult for many patients. The difficulty and expense of a trip to Germany for someone disabled from MS discouraged many patients from even considering trying it.

Having great compassion for the struggles of low-income people and people with disabling health disorders such as MS, I began an intense and earnest search for any other alternative approaches that might help MS patients. The recent access to the Internet expanded my ability to review both published research studies and anecdotal reports on various supplements that had helped some MS patients. I wrote about these various discoveries in the library's quarterly newsletter.

One day in the fall of 1999, I was reading a newsletter, *Positive Health News*, that our library received, which published anecdotal reports of various natural supplements or protocols that reportedly benefited AIDS patients. http://www.keephopealive.org/report19.html

The newsletter contained an article by Bernard Bihari, MD, who was having some success treating AIDS patients with an off-label treatment called Low Dose Naltrexone (LDN). The article also mentioned his work using LDN to help people with many autoimmune disorders.

I was very excited to speak with Dr. Bihari about his work with autoimmune disorders and was not disappointed with his initial and continuing welcoming responses to my many questions.

I was calling him almost weekly to inquire about the range of conditions that might be helped by LDN and asked him about his results with patients. He was always open and sharing of his experiences with his patients. My inquiries ranged far beyond MS, although that was my initial primary interest.

Early on in our conversations, Dr. Bihari told me about the first MS patient he had suggested try LDN. He obtained permission from her to give me her phone number, so I could speak with her about her experience. Although she admitted that she was not always consistent about taking it every day, she conveyed with enthusiasm the benefits she believed she derived from taking LDN for several years after her MS diagnosis.

I wrote about her story in the library's quarterly newsletter, adding LDN as an approach for MS patients to consider. Over the next 20 years I was able to watch LDN continue to grow in use from a grassroots approach for people with MS and other autoimmune disorders who were desperate for better health. Slowly the message reached more and more people, until now many thousands of people with various health disorders are reporting benefits from it. Even now, most of the physicians who use LDN are considered alternative-minded physicians. It took almost ten years before I saw it being written about in one of the leading health publications our library subscribed to, Dr. Julian Whittaker's newsletter.

I was immensely delighted to be an early part of this growing community that started from Dr. Bihari's medical understanding of low endorphin levels in both AIDS patients and patients with other health disorders that might be remedied with very low doses of naltrexone.

My understanding of the potential of LDN for various health disorders grew with every conversation I had with Dr. Bihari over several years. He would usually be too busy to talk with me during the day when he was seeing patients, so he would call me back at home on Friday evenings after his work week was over. He would be munching on one of those fabulous New York sandwiches while we chatted. Friday night phone calls with Dr. Bihari quickly became one of my favorite times of the week.

I soon developed a profound respect and deep fondness for this wonderful doctor who was so generous with his knowledge, time, energy, and experience. During the 20 years I worked at the Brewer Science Library, I have called many doctors to follow up on their innovative therapies. Many of them were willing to talk honestly about their experiences with patients during one or two phone calls. None were like Dr. Bihari. He was very special to me and still is. Over two or three years I probably spoke with him a hundred times. I treasure all our many conversations.

Passing on the information about LDN to people whose lives might be improved by using it was truly the highlight of my work in the alternative health field.

The majority of calls to the library were from MS patients seeking information about Dr. Nieper's Ca-EAP treatment. I also shared with them the potential of LDN, either as an inexpensive therapy to try first or in combination with Ca-EAP. Several patients who had obtained significant health improvement on Ca-

EAP therapy added LDN therapy to their comprehensive approach for optimal health. Some felt it further benefited them, and some did not. Some MS patients decided to try the easy and inexpensive LDN therapy first and benefited so significantly that they did not pursue any other treatment.

LDN has resulted in many dramatic reductions or remissions of health issues for many people. Some people—who have not realized as much benefit as they hoped for—should consider adding other strategies to their LDN protocol. For instance:

- eating a healthy diet with many vegetables
- eating little to no sugar
- doing a three- to four-month trial of gluten-free eating
- doing the same trial of dairy-free eating
- reducing stress as much as possible
- exercising as able
- practicing gratitude
- fostering good relationships

Treatments some patients with MS have found helpful, either alone or with LDN: a fat-soluble B1, such as benfotiamine (http://www.mwt.net/~drbrewer/benfotiamine.htm); or histamine therapy (http://www.goodshape.net); or gold therapy (http://www.mwt.net/~drbrewer/Gold_Regeneration.htm). And some post-menopausal female MS patients have benefited from natural hormone therapy and low doses of DHEA.

On the other hand, I have spoken to many people who have incorporated all these other healthy beneficial strategies who did not get their health situation to turn around until they started on

LDN, because LDN provides a specific interaction their bodies respond to.

Obtaining LDN was quite problematic in the beginning when I was first talking and writing about it, and still is for some people. Bringing LDN information to their general practitioners turned out to be the best strategy for obtaining a prescription. Specialists were much less likely to prescribe anything outside of the standard of care.

The most innovative and inexpensive approach to obtaining LDN was posted on Fritz Bell's www.Goodshape.net website. People could get the 50 mg pressed tablets, dissolve them in 50 ml of distilled water, and easily and cheaply obtain a solution that provided 1 mg per 1 ml of solution, enabling them to use a baby syringe to target a dosage within the 1 to 4.5 mg range. Presently the India-based pharmacy, www.alldaychemist.com, still offers a 10-pill packet of naltrexone for about $20. One box of 10 pressed tablets provides approximately six months of use taken at 3 mg a day. For those able to obtain a prescription, Skip's Pharmacy offers a very reasonable price.

Over the years I came across only two or three people who reacted negatively to LDN usage, even at a very low dose of 1 mg a day. That reaction was very unusual, though. MS patients are often very sensitive, and Dr. Bihari suggested that they initiate LDN therapy at a low dose of 1 mg to 1.5 mg and gradually, over weeks or even months, increase it to 3 mg taken nightly before bed. Some MS patients did well at dosages somewhere between 3 to 4.5 mg, but many found the most benefit at 3 mg.

Dr. Bihari also treated patients with various cancers that responded positively to LDN. He shared his experience with me about an AIDS patient who developed lymphoma and experienced a remission from that cancer on LDN. This led to many phone calls from me about various cancers to find out if he had used LDN with any patients with those cancers.

Many men with prostate cancer called me, requesting information about alternative approaches. Dr. Bihari shared with me that he had treated two men with prostate cancer who responded positively to LDN. They had not previously undergone hormone therapy as the majority of men had. Dr. Bihari postulated that the hormone therapy might have changed the prostate's cellular membrane's response to endorphins. Many people with various types of cancers have added LDN to their protocols, hoping for the positive response that others have obtained.

With some embarrassment, I even called him about how to treat a dog with LDN, but he handled it like any other call and figured out the dosage to use based on the dog's weight.

Over the years, I have been delighted to see that hundreds of doctors throughout the world now prescribe LDN. Most of them prescribe it for the conditions Dr. Bihari used it for with his patients: autoimmune diseases; some cancers; and some neurodegenerative diseases, such as Parkinson's, MS, autism, post-polio syndrome, and others.

But, as other doctors became aware of his work, some of them tried LDN on patients that Dr. Bihari might not have seen in his practice. One of the doctors who experimented with a unique use of LDN was diabetic expert Richard Bernstein, MD. He found that LDN did not impact his patients' blood sugar levels or their diabetes. However, it did help some of his patients to experience a reduction in the strong carbohydrate cravings that made staying on a healthy low-carbohydrate diet very difficult. The amount of LDN that helped was unique to each patient; some were taking 1 mg or less in the afternoon when the craving was the strongest. Others took it at night in various low doses, and it helped to control their cravings the next day. Considering the present and growing epidemic of diabetes, this use of LDN is something diabetics might want to investigate.

I believe Dr. Bihari would have been delighted by the influence his discovery has attained and is still realizing, even after his death.

As a man, Dr. Bihari was kind, generous, enthusiastic, highly intelligent, interesting, and very willing to share his knowledge and understanding. As a doctor, he discovered a simple and inexpensive therapy that has been health- and life-transforming for many people. I feel honored to have played a small part in helping to get his information out to a needy public.

Like Fritz Bell, Christina White learned about LDN nearly 20 years ago. Christina was so impressed by LDN, and by the man who literally invented it, that she decided to write about and champion it to others. Had she not done that, I doubt that LDN would have become as well-known as it now is. As I wrote in my introduction to her chapter, I am surprised that Christina hasn't been interviewed about LDN before this; I am honored to have her represented here.

CHAPTER 5

How Frank Melhus Found Healing with Low Dose Naltrexone and Shared It with the World

I am particularly excited that Frank Melhus has agreed to tell his story for our book. Frank's name is not widely known outside of his native Norway, but his accomplishments are legendary throughout the LDN community. Frank was so indebted to LDN for saving him from near-blindness that he resolved to use his position as a documentarian for TV2, the most prominent commercial television network in Norway, to share his own LDN success story.

After the documentary aired in 2013, the use of LDN in Norway increased 500 percent—almost overnight. Even more amazing: 75 percent of general practitioners in Norway now prescribe LDN.

News about Frank's documentary also spread to the entire LDN community outside of Norway, all thanks to Frank's persistence, brilliance, and passion.

We hope that, by sharing Frank's inspiring story, other documentary filmmakers around the world will follow suit. These stories of real people's successes with LDN—people like those featured in Frank's documentary, and people like those who share their stories in this book—can spread the word most effectively. LDN is a "people's movement," and what better way to reach real people than through the media?

Here, in Frank's words, is his story.

I began working at TV2—the largest commercial channel in Norway—in 1993. For the first 22 years I was a videographer, and since then, a producer.

It is strange to me that I've become such an advocate for LDN. You see, I was always against what I considered "unproven" treatments like LDN. I called them "voodoo." I was the first guy to run to a medical doctor to get pills. Whenever I visited the United States, I was always going to the pharmacy to get pills. You have such great drugs in the US!

I have been sick a lot in my life. From the time I was a teenager, I was in bed for two weeks every autumn, and again every winter, with a temperature of 40° Celsius (104° Fahrenheit). And over time I developed several autoimmune symptoms.

The first health problem I noticed was when working out I had trouble breathing. It was some type of asthma that affected my lungs when I was doing strenuous workouts. I also started getting pain in my joints. I learned I was "HLA Positive"—the gene commonly associated with ankylosing spondylitis. My mother has that gene as well. When I started getting the intense joint inflammation, my doctor thought it was the start of spondylitis.

In 2011, I was home sick for almost six months. I had no strength; I was so tired I couldn't get up, and I was very depressed. That didn't make sense to me because I have a great family and so many good things in my life.

Over the next six months, I got my strength back more or less, and I was intending to start working again after my summer holidays. But a few days before my wife and I were going to have a big celebration with family and friends for our joint fortieth birthdays, I started noticing that something was wrong with my left eye. It was painful and felt as if there was something in front of it, making my vision a bit blurry.

At first, I didn't think much about it, but then it started hurting more, so I went to my doctor, who sent me to a specialist. The optic neurologist said I had optic neuritis—an inflammation of the nerve in the eye—an autoimmune condition. He was worried and told me this could be serious. He sent me directly to the hospital where I had an MRI of my brain. Earlier, though, I Googled "optic neuritis" and found out that there was a 50 percent chance that I would develop multiple sclerosis within five years. That made me very nervous.

The MRI didn't disclose anything, but the doctor told me, "If you get a lot worse you should come back." However, he rescheduled me for an appointment in two weeks. The next day, my eye became a little bit worse, and one day before the big party I woke up to find that I was blind in my left eye.

I couldn't see anything. I had been sleeping, and the room was very dark when I woke up, and I turned the lights on, and I thought, "What happened?" When I closed my right eye, there was total blackness. It was like I had become totally blind in the course of one night. I freaked out, so my wife took me to the hospital. The attack was so severe that they put me on a very high-dose intravenous steroid drip. They said there was nothing else they could do, but the steroids might cool down the attack. I went home. We had the party, but I was very concerned about my health.

My right eye was normal. The left was totally blind. My doctor said there was nothing that could be done. All he said was: "You might get MS, you might not."

But being a videographer, my vision and eyesight are crucial to me. I started staying at home, feeling sick, doing research. I thought I would try to see what was out there, and I typed in "autoimmune/MS alternative treatments."

I found a small article titled "Low Dose Naltrexone (LDN)" on a Norwegian website. At first, I thought LDN was just more voodoo. As I read about this "miracle drug," I assumed that if it were the real deal, my doctor would have used it on me. If LDN worked the way these patients were saying, it would be in every hospital, and available to any patient everywhere. In other words, I didn't believe the claims about LDN.

But then I remembered a rule we follow all the time in investigative journalism. It is a very good rule: "Follow the money!"

I discovered that LDN was inexpensive, so there was no money to be made from it. I wondered why—if there is no money in it—do some doctors still endorse and recommend it? Then I thought: "Okay, maybe there could be something here." I did more research and started to think maybe this was something I should try.

I decided to talk to Steinar Hauge, the creator of the Norwegian LDN website located at https://sites.google.com/view/ldnno/startside. He is an MS patient and champion of LDN. He invited me to visit him.

I went to see him, and we had a coffee, six weeks after I had gone blind in my left eye. He told me everything he knew about LDN and said, "If you are going to try to get a prescription for LDN, be aware that your doctor might hesitate to prescribe it for you because there are not many people using it in Norway—maybe only a few hundred."

Earlier that Monday when I visited Steinar, I had seen the chief eye specialist in the hospital, where I had regular Monday appointments. For six weeks, I had been having photos taken of the optic nerve in my blind eye, along with the other, healthy eye for comparison.

On this Monday there was no difference; there had been no change to the optic nerve in the photo. My left eye was still very inflamed. "You have to prepare yourself that your eyesight will be severely damaged forever," the doctor said.

But, by that time I had begun to be able to see a little bit: If someone was sitting in front of a window, I could see his or her outline, and I could almost guess who it was. But the progress was very, very slow. It had been six weeks, and at this point, there had been almost no progress at all.

After meeting Steinar, I called my primary care doctor, an excellent practitioner, and got an appointment that same day. At the appointment, I told her, "You've got to help me. I am more or less blind in my left eye, and at the hospital, they say they can't do anything for me. I would like to try this drug called Low Dose Naltrexone."

She looked it up, and said: "Okay, it exists in 50 milligrams, but is used for alcohol addiction or as an antidote for opiates."

I explained to her about the research I had been doing, but she still didn't want to write the prescription. I called Steinar Hauge while I was sitting in her office, and I asked her to talk to him. She did, and then she asked him if he knew any neurologists who were prescribing LDN. He mentioned the name of one neurologist she was familiar with, Dr. Halfdan Kierulfand. Then she said, "Okay, I will write you a prescription." Success! (I later interviewed Dr. Kierulfand for the documentary.)

I filled the prescription and decided I would start that same evening. But that day I was beginning to feel strange. I don't know how to describe it, but I found myself not being able to stand up. And I started sweating. Something was not right.

I got a friend to drive me to the ER. They did some initial tests. Although they didn't find anything, they kept me there overnight. I called my wife at work, and told her, "Before you come to the hospital I need you to go home and pick up this very small box of pills on the kitchen table. I want to start taking them tonight."

I was in observation, sitting in a room and being checked every three hours, when my wife walked in with the box of LDN tablets.

I took the first pill, a 3 mg dosage. I was freaked out because I didn't know how I would react to the drug. I didn't have any dramatic expectations that it would be a "miracle" drug. But, still, I had a small amount of hope.

The next morning when I woke up, I felt different. I'm not sure how to describe it, but I had been feeling very weak and depressed for a long time. But now, suddenly, it was like someone had turned the power on. Since the hospital couldn't find anything on the exams, they sent me home.

For the first time in about nine months, I found myself laughing. I was watching some stupid television show, and I started laughing. I was enjoying myself. I hadn't done that for such a long time. I felt good things begin to happen in my body. The energy was coming back, and my mood was improving. It took less than 24 hours for me to feel the change. I thought, "Wow! Is this just a placebo? What's happening?" I felt great, and the following week I could tell I was picking up, with small improvements.

But, there was one problem: My left eye was getting worse.

I had this test at home where I would look at the blinds in front of the window. Before I started taking the LDN, I could see some details with the blinds, but suddenly I couldn't see them anymore. It was almost like I was backsliding. That freaked me out. "You're so stupid," I thought. "Why did you have to try this LDN? Maybe this wasn't so smart."

I called Steinar, and he said this is quite a normal response from the body. He told me that it might take a few days, maybe even a week, for my immune system to calm down; that LDN could aggravate the immune system at first. But he said that soon, it should calm down. So, I continued to take the pills. I would trust him. I would stay on the LDN.

Then it was Monday again. I was back at the hospital getting more pictures taken of both eyes, the seventh time I had been there.

On all the other Mondays there had been no visual difference in the optic nerve in my left eye. It had been very inflamed. The right eye was always normal. Each week, they showed me the images, using the right eye as a reference.

But *this* Monday, although my eyesight was worse than it had been before I started LDN, my body felt better than it had in years. As the lab assistant took the pictures, I was sitting up close, opposite her desk, and as she was looking at them she said, "Shit! What's happened here?"

And I said, "Do you mean that in a good way or a bad way?" And she said, "Come see for yourself."

She showed me the images, and she said, "This is the right eye, which is healthy, and this was last week's photo (which I recognized), and this is your left eye today." I said, "No, you've mixed up the right eye and the left eye."

"No," she said, "this is your left eye. It looks completely normal. What have you been doing?" I said, "Uh, nothing." I was concerned that, if I told her about the LDN, she would tell the optic neurologist and he would insist that I stop taking it. So, I said, "I didn't do anything."

I had previously discussed LDN with my optic neurologist, and he had said, "There is no way you're getting this drug here." He had thought it was just hearsay, and that there was no science behind it. There was no way I would be getting the drug from him. I knew he was opposed to it.

I went home and thought, "This is some serious drug, having this kind of effect in just seven days!" Steinar was right.

Within about four weeks, my eyesight in my left eye was more or less normal. When it started to heal, it happened quite quickly. Today I have 100 percent normal eyesight in both eyes.

In the weeks after starting LDN, I felt all my autoimmune symptoms disappear. My asthma was gone, my joint problems were gone. And I have not had any symptoms since then. I haven't even had a cold.

I totally turned around. I haven't taken another pill in the last six years—just LDN. I used to have headaches about once a week maybe. I haven't had one in six years. And I've changed as a person because I was very pro conventional medicine, and regular drugs. Now I am very opposed. I have more faith in treatments that are more natural and that don't cost a lot of money.

I had another appointment with the optic neurologist while I was regaining my sight, and I told him about the LDN. I thought if I talked to him now, he couldn't take it away from me. But he wouldn't listen.

"Look at the images that your assistant took!" I said. "In one week, my eye healed. That's not interesting to you?" He didn't even look at me. He said, "We don't do that here."

This was very disheartening, but that's when I got my big idea. I thought, "Okay, I work in the media. I could reach a lot of people. I *have* to tell the public the story about this drug, which no doctor wants to prescribe. But there is *something* about this drug that's useful."

I talked to my boss. I told her my story and said I thought we should tell the story about this medication because it could help many people. She was difficult to convince because the biggest problem with LDN is that there is not much research behind it. That's what you always hear.

"Never mind the science," I told her. "There will never be science on this drug because there is no money to be made from it. But, couldn't we tell the story anyway? Couldn't we say there isn't a lot of science behind this, but the patients say their experience is that it has helped them?"

So that's what we did. We created a documentary that tells patients' stories from their viewpoints. It's not investigative journalism.

It was one of the first documentaries we made for the series, "Vårt Lille Land" ("Our Small Country"). And my boss, who had initially been so skeptical, eventually became the editor for this documentary, which was titled "Unknown Medicine." My good colleague, Kaare Skard, was the reporter on the documentary, and he put a great deal of hard work into it.

Through the small LDN community in Norway, we found a woman named Nansy Schulzki, with multiple sclerosis, who agreed to be featured in the documentary. We also needed to find some doctors who prescribe LDN, to hear their stories. We went to Dublin to interview the wonderful Dr. Edmond O'Flaherty, who is a strong advocate of LDN. He listens to his patients.

Making the documentary was easy because we had the connections and the resources to tell it. I would love to follow up further on the progress of some of these patients. That was missing from this documentary. But, we had so little time to produce it. We were working on several projects at the same time and had about three months from start to finish.

The day the LDN show aired, I was sitting at home, and my wife was traveling. I was alone in my living room, and I thought, "Wow, we actually got it on the air! I am one of the most powerful people in medicine in Norway, today, at this very moment!"

I knew this was getting out there, and that it would be good for so many people. That felt really, really good.

Our documentary about LDN was the most viewed story that year. It is now online in the original Norwegian; there is also a version with English subtitles online as well. https://www.youtube.com/watch?v=rBd2gv8UGU0

When the film was broadcast, people started calling. There was an explosion in membership in the LDN Norge (LDN Norway) Facebook group https://www.facebook.com/groups/262889817077593. Before the documentary aired there had been 200 people in the group. After one week, its membership had grown to 5,000. [Author's Note: Today, it is at over 11,000.]

There was a tsunami of LDN prescriptions. One of the great things was that our news department kept following the story, talking to new patients, as well as to doctors. The neurologists in Norway were very angry with us because we told the story. The head of the neurology department at the biggest hospital in Oslo stopped by. She was interviewed and said that no patients should use LDN because it is unproven and could be dangerous, along with everything else she could think of to persuade people not to take it.

The interview was broadcast and shared on the station's website. Steinar had told me about this woman and said that she is a professor and that she teaches new medical students. He said that whenever she mentions LDN to them, she tells them that it is an unproven drug. "You should never prescribe this drug to a patient."

But I knew that now the word was out, and more than a tenth of the population had seen the program. And the word was spreading in the multiple sclerosis community. It was a good feeling that the story was out there. It was like a snowball starting to roll and get bigger as it rolls, or a train that is impossible to stop.

There are now 15,000 patients with MS and other diseases taking LDN in Norway, and a Norwegian medical journal even published an article in 2017 about the LDN phenomenon started by the documentary. It had the gratifying title, "A Sudden and Unprecedented Increase in Low Dose Naltrexone (LDN) Prescribing in Norway." https://munin.uit.no/bitstream/handle/10037/10400/article.pdf

At first, when the show aired, and people showed up at their doctor's offices demanding to get a prescription, most doctors refused. They said, "We don't do that here." There were quite a few medical centers with groups of doctors, and they had meetings and agreed that they should not prescribe LDN.

Initially, lots of people on Facebook and people who contacted Steinar were reporting that they weren't able to get a prescription.

But with time, people were showing up with great results, and I am happy to report that many of these doctors turned around. Now, some even suggest that their patients try LDN. Almost everyone in Norway who wants a prescription for LDN will actually get it. And within the last year, if your doctor prescribes LDN for you, you can get it at almost no cost. You pay a very small amount, and the government pays for the rest.

While our documentary was wildly successful, looking back, I think the ideal story would be to follow people with three or four different conditions from the start of their illness. You would film them while they are sick and not getting the help or the relief they need from their regular medications. Then, you would follow them, and see how they progress. That was my initial plan for this documentary as well, but there was too little time.

The success of LDN and our documentary has changed my life, both personally and professionally. For one thing, I no longer shun the so-called "alternative" therapies. As a matter of fact, it is the expensive, toxic pharmaceuticals—which I used to be so fond of—that I stay away from now. I feel blessed to have been able to tell the LDN story here in Norway, and—thanks to the Internet—our documentary has been seen by nearly a million people worldwide. LDN is definitely a "people's movement." It's truly "people-powered medicine."

∽

I hope that sharing Frank's story of how he went from grateful patient to LDN documentarian will inspire other filmmakers to follow in his footsteps. As Frank's account demonstrates, there is no better way to bolster a "people's movement" like LDN than by telling patient success stories through the media.

CHAPTER 6

How Suffering with MS Turned Linda Elsegood into an LDN Hero: A Tribute to Persistence

I've known Linda Elsegood since 2009 when a group of us met on Skype to plan for the first International Low Dose Naltrexone Awareness Week in October of that year. Her UK-based charity, the LDN Research Trust, was just five years old at the time, but she was already known as a formidable advocate for LDN. Linda told her story in Chapter 12 of Honest Medicine, *and is sharing it here again, in expanded form.*

When you read about how Linda turned great suffering into advocacy for others, you'll understand why she has an important place in this book, as well.

Here is Linda's story.

∽

I was diagnosed with multiple sclerosis (MS) in August 2000, when I was 44 years old. However, I had symptoms many years earlier, starting with bladder problems when I was 17.

My most serious symptoms began in 1988 when I was 32.

I was very, very sick. I had numbness and pins and needles that came and went. When I'd tell my doctor that my calf muscle in my right leg would go numb, he'd tell me I had a slipped disc. When I told him that I had electric shocks down to my fingertips when I put my chin down, he'd say it was a trapped nerve in my neck and suggested I wear a collar. But my husband worked, and I had children who were involved in various activities. We lived in a village in the middle of nowhere, so I had to drive—and you can't drive safely while wearing a collar. So, I didn't do that.

I had double vision, too, which made life almost unbearable. I could see fine out of each eye separately, but my two eyes could not work together. So, I wore an eye patch over one eye for a few hours and then swapped it to the other eye. That way, I was still working both eyes, but individually, not together.

My hearing was also affected. I couldn't hear anything at all out of my left ear. It was totally dead. According to the technician who administered my hearing test, it is very unusual not to hear anything at all out of an ear. But I didn't.

My worst symptom was brain fog. If you haven't had it, you can't begin to understand how hard it can be. Just trying to hold a conversation was next to impossible. I couldn't recall vocabulary, I got words muddled, and it was a struggle to piece a sentence together. It was as if English wasn't my first language. I would try to think of a word, and it would make sense to me. I knew what I wanted to say, but what actually came out of my mouth was something totally different. It was as if I was suffering from Alzheimer's. I just couldn't say what I wanted to say. That was the scariest, most frightening thing.

If I spent too long trying to put together what I wanted to say, I'd fall asleep! People would be talking to me, I'd be trying to listen and process the information they were telling me, and I'd fall asleep! It was SO difficult to communicate with people.

It seemed like my husband Marc was always correcting me. He'd say, "That's wrong," or "That's not tea, it's coffee; you called it tea." I'd say, "Well, you know I don't drink tea, and you know I meant coffee." He'd say, "I know. But if I correct you, you'll remember for next time."

But it didn't work like that. I didn't remember for the next time. It was depressing to even open my mouth because I was always told I was wrong, and that was really hard. And because I also had chronic fatigue, the effort of trying to sort things out with this fog in my brain was impossible. I was slurring my speech, as though I'd had a stroke. I had to chew my food carefully. But I'd still start to choke on it. People had to pound me on the back.

The only saving grace was that I slept 20 hours a day! If I was awake for four hours, I had done well. And it wasn't four hours at a time—it would be maybe 20 minutes here, half an hour there—that kind of thing.

I had no balance, either, which meant I would spend a lot of time on the floor. I would trip and fall and stumble over nothing. I had to "furniture walk." By that I mean I'd walk holding onto furniture or walls to try to give myself a bit of balance. I remember being told by the doctor, "If you go out and feel one of these vertigo dizzy spells coming on, you must lie down—whether you are in a supermarket, or in the street—lie down! Because you're going to fall anyway, and if you lie down before you fall, you're less likely to hurt yourself." So that is what I did. But I didn't go out very often, so I didn't have to disgrace myself by doing that. Things got so bad that I was often in a wheelchair.

I remember one day we had friends coming, and I was in the hall. My head started spinning, so I just lay down exactly where I was. The friends rang the doorbell, and my husband said, "Come in. Oh, don't mind Linda," and he stepped over me. Our friends were horrified! "Aren't you going to help her? Why are you leaving her lying there?" And he said, "She gets up when she feels she can, but right now she's got to lie on the floor." As I said, they were horrified.

I had problems with my bowels as well. It was bowels, bladder, slurred speech, brain fog, and restless legs.

Of course, in hindsight, these were all MS symptoms. Once I got the diagnosis, I could see that I had had MS for a long time.

Even before I was diagnosed, I was given a course of intravenous steroids, which did absolutely nothing for me. Six weeks later, the neurologist was very concerned. I had optic neuritis on top of all my other symptoms, and my double vision was really bad. The neurologist said he was worried that I was going to become blind and deaf, and he wanted to give me another course of intravenous steroids. The prospect of being deaf and blind was very scary, so I took the intravenous steroids. In a few weeks, they started to work very slightly, but I wasn't anywhere near back to normal.

By August 2000, just before my diagnosis, I was in the hospital. The nurse came in to draw my blood—I'd already had 20-odd different blood tests to try and determine what was wrong with me—and she said, "So, how long have you had multiple sclerosis?" I said, "I haven't got MS." By the way she looked at me, I *knew* I had MS. She said, "Oh, I'm sorry. I was thinking of another patient. I got you confused."

But then a few hours later the neurologist told me I had MS.

After the second course of steroids, I asked my doctor, "How long do you think it will be before I start feeling better?" He said, "Well, to be honest, I think if you were going to feel better, you would have done so by now."

I was often in terrible pain—pain so excruciating that it would make me vomit; so bad I couldn't see. I was taking really strong painkillers. They made me nauseous—like morning sickness, travel sickness, and motion sickness all combined. When I moved my head, I felt like I was going to throw up. I would have to think to myself, before I took them, "Which is worse, the pain or nausea?" The medication didn't take the pain away completely. I could still feel it, but it was bearable. When I felt I couldn't stand it anymore,

I would take the painkillers, but I'd have to lie perfectly still and not move my head. Then I'd wish I hadn't taken them.

The only actual MS drug I was offered was Rebif. I took it for eight months. The needles were like fishing hooks. They were bent, so when they went in, they really hurt! Also, my body reacted to the preservative in the prefilled syringes. So, every time I was injected, it felt like I'd been stung by a bee. It was so painful!

Since I was having so many problems with my bladder and my bowels, I went to see a gastroenterologist. She tested my blood and asked, "What are you doing? What are you taking?" I told her I was taking Rebif, and she said, "And your neurologist knows this?" I said, "Yes." And she said, "It's killing you—it's doing irreversible damage to your liver!" She said she would talk with my neurologist.

When I saw my neurologist, I told him I wouldn't take Rebif anymore.

I wasn't really living. I was just surviving. There was nothing else that I was being offered.

In 2003, I went to see the neurologist and told him I couldn't live like this. He examined me and told me to sit down. He held his hand out to shake mine, and said, "I'm really sorry to tell you, you have secondary progressive MS now." He let go of my hand, opened the door, and said, "There's nothing more we can do for you."

I was devastated. I contemplated ending it all—more for my family than for me. I felt I was stopping everybody from having a normal life, whatever that is! But I didn't want my 15-year-old daughter to find me, so I didn't kill myself. I knew I had to do something.

I was desperate to find something that was going to help me. I knew I couldn't be unique—that there must be other people with MS, who were doing *something* and were feeling better. I was on a mission to find the "something" that would help me, and I didn't care what it was because the doctors weren't offering me anything. I sat at the computer and started to research online. But, with a patch over one eye, I could only be online for a few minutes at a time. So, on my many trips to the toilet, which were very frequent while I was awake, I would sit at the computer for ten minutes at a time. After ten minutes I just couldn't process anything.

I learn about LDN!

One day, I managed to find some people in the US who were using LDN, and they were willing to talk to me. Everybody agreed that if it didn't do me any good it wasn't going to do me any harm, either.

It took me several weeks to really research LDN. I found Dr. Bob Lawrence in Wales, who was prescribing LDN, and I had a chat with him. He sent me information to print out and take to my doctor. I took it to her, and she said she wasn't a partner in the practice, but she would get them to look at it. She told me to come back in two weeks, which I did. She said they had reviewed the information but were not prepared to prescribe LDN. She said that if it were her, she would try LDN; and if I could find a doctor to prescribe it for me, she would monitor me. So, Dr. Lawrence prescribed it for me, and my doctor monitored me.

I started the LDN, and I didn't have any side effects at all. I was actually disappointed. People don't like the side effects of drugs, but I *wanted* side effects. I'd been told that I'd probably have vivid dreams. I might have constipation. I might have worsening of pre-existing symptoms. I just wanted to know it was working. I wanted *something* to happen. If I had side effects, it would show that it was doing something. But I had no side effects at all. I didn't give up, though, and I carried on taking it. I thought to myself that this was my last chance at trying to become "me" again. But I was afraid it wasn't going to work.

Then, presto! It was such a surprise when three weeks later, things started to improve. I woke up one morning, and it was as though somebody had adjusted a television set that wasn't tuned in properly. (People who are used to the new televisions won't know what I'm talking about, but years ago television sets had to be tuned in.) I slowly began to see and hear. My balance returned. My bladder and bowels settled down. I started to feel like "me" again.

I still know I have MS—I'm not saying I'm cured, and there are times when I am really aware of my MS symptoms, especially when I get a cold or the flu or a chest infection. There are many people who say that on LDN they no longer get infections. I do. Anything that's going around, I get it! And stress does make things worse, like when my mom had a heart attack—and years later, when she died.

While the fog in my head cleared in three weeks, the other symptoms—mainly the restless legs—took longer to disappear. You know, the burning limbs where you feel that you're on fire, as though you've been out in the sun—like you're sunburned and can't cool down your limbs. But when I actually touched my legs, they felt cold. They weren't burning. But inside, they felt as if they were on fire. Finally, that went away, and the numbness and the pins and needles left, along with the twitching muscles. After taking LDN, as time went on, my legs started slowly to move less and less in bed, and I was able to get more rest.

I must say, if I hadn't found LDN when I did, I don't think I'd be here today.

I am able to achieve things now, and that's a really big thing for me. I'm a workaholic. I love to set challenges for myself and achieve them. When you can't do that—when you can't achieve anything, and you can't control your bladder, which is something a two-year-old can do—you disappoint yourself on so many different levels.

To be able to have control over so many different things again is tremendous.

Life after LDN

Now that I was feeling so much better, was I going to say, "I'm okay," and carry on with my life? I decided I had to tell others who had heard the devastating words, "There's nothing more we can do for you," that, indeed, there *is* something they can do for themselves. And there is a good chance that that "something"—LDN—will help them like it helped me.

I wanted to help other people escape from that deep dark place where I had been. First, I had a meeting with the MS Society and was referred to a neurologist they worked with. His advice was, "If you want to do anything, nobody is going to take you seriously unless you are a registered charity." So, he gave me the task of setting up a charity. Frankly, I think he believed I would fail—that I would give up and go away.

It took me five months, but I finally got charity status! I've never had a challenge like it. I like a challenge. I spoke to just about everybody at the Charity Commission office, the organization that regulates charities in England and Wales.[55] I think they set up hurdles for me to fail. But I wasn't going to fail. I would fill out their forms, and they would send the forms back to me, with notations such as "You can't do this," "You can't do that," "This needs changing." And I would send it back the same day by recorded delivery [Author's Note: "recorded delivery" is UK English for certified mail], and I'd phone to check that they'd gotten it—even though I knew by the tracking that they had—asking when I would get a reply. And they would say, "It's been scheduled for three weeks from now." Then when one department was happy with what I was doing, it would be passed on to another department, and the whole process would start all over again. Over that five-month period, I think I probably even spoke to the cleaning staff at some point because I had talked to just about everybody!

There were challenges even after getting our charity status, though. For instance, you're not allowed to promote an unlicensed drug. You can only raise awareness. There is a fine line between the two, but you're not allowed to promote in any way whatsoever. So, that's what we do: raise awareness about LDN.

We chose the name the LDN Research Trust. We put up our website at www.ldnresearchtrust.org. It has a tremendous amount of information. And we have a newsletter and a forum. From the beginning, we found that there was a lot of interest in LDN. The phone never stopped ringing. It still hasn't. Recently, after 13 years, the forum was closed, since most people use the LDN Research Trust Facebook page at https://www.facebook.com/groups/LDNRT.

In 2009, we started putting on conferences devoted to LDN. Between 2009 and 2017, we've held conferences both in the US (Palatine, IL; Las Vegas NV; Orlando, FL; and Portland, OR) and in the United Kingdom (Birmingham, England). So far, we have two more planned: one for 2018 in Glasgow, Scotland, and another for 2019 in Portland. We plan to have more conferences in future years.

We've had speakers from all over the world and from many different medical specialties speak at and attend our conferences. Speakers include doctors, compounding pharmacists and patients. They've spoken about their successes using LDN for all kinds of conditions, autoimmune and non-autoimmune alike.[56] Dr. Burt Berkson has spoken, as have Dr. Phil Boyle (infertility), Dr. Mark Shukhman (psychiatry), Dr. Preedap Chopra (pain), Drs. Akbar Khan and Angus Dalgleish (cancer), and Dr. Brian Udell (autism), to name just a very few. And gastroenterologist Dr. Leonard

Weinstock is always looking at other conditions LDN might help.[57] [Author's Note: All the conferences, along with many of the speakers, are listed in the Appendix.]

People can attend, either in person or on the computer via streaming video. We realize that wherever we hold a conference, not everybody will be happy with the location. Since we have members all around the world, only a certain number of people can attend in person. But since our conferences are all live-streamed, you can watch them live from anywhere in the world. If you miss a presentation because of the time difference, the videos are all stored online—some for free, and others for a nominal fee.

We were very blessed at the 2017 conference that most of the administrators from our Facebook group came to volunteer! One even came from New Zealand. And of course, they didn't get paid. They paid their own way to come and help. Our aim is to make the conferences bigger every year.

In addition to the conferences, I've interviewed over 700 people so far—prescribing doctors, compounding pharmacists, and patients—in both audio and video formats. They, too, are online. And now, we have the LDN Radio Show, located online at LDNRadio.org, which has been a tremendous success.

The LDN Research Trust has produced three documentaries so far: The first two are titled "The LDN Story";[58] and "LDN & Cancer: The Game Changer."[59] The third is about Lyme disease. All our documentaries are available free, online, on our Vimeo channel, located at http://www.vimeo.com/ldnresearchtrust. The Lyme project is phenomenal. There is so much misinformation out there about Lyme. We have gathered a number of Lyme-literate experts. Because everybody has so much crucial information to share, we have featured the best information from each expert in the hour-long documentary. We also have a "docuseries" with a half-hour video from each speaker. [Author's Note: You may watch the Lyme disease documentary, "Bullseye: Low Dose Naltrexone and Lyme Disease," at https://www.ldnresearchtrust.org/Lyme-Disease-LDN-Documentary.]

Another project, *The LDN Book*,[60] published by Chelsea Green, was launched at our 2016 conference in Orlando. It contains seven chapters written by physicians who have experienced excellent results prescribing LDN for their patients, as well as a chapter by a compounding pharmacist, and another by two LDN cancer researchers. I am happy to report that the book, available worldwide, has gotten excellent reviews.

The Research Trust's most recent project is the LDN App, a health tracker app[61] free to patients, which was launched in March of 2018. It works on smartphones—both iPhones and Androids—as well as on tablets, PCs, and Macs. This app helps physicians and pharmacists monitor their patients who are taking LDN; and allows patients to track their medications, their mood, their pain and their exercise. Jill Brook, a researcher, has been a tremendous help with this project. We don't know actual patients' details—they are just ID numbers. The important point is that the patient controls which doctors and pharmacists—if any—they want to have access to their private information. And if they change their mind, and don't want a doctor or pharmacist to track them anymore, they just remove that practitioner's license number, and it's like a door being closed. They can't access that patient's information anymore. The patients—and this is important—are ultimately responsible for who has access to their data.

We have a very busy private Facebook group, with over 26,000 members and an LDN Research Trust forum. We also have some wonderful volunteers, helping me in several different ways. For instance, some volunteers help with doctors' requests. That's a big thing. We can put pharmacists' names and contact information on our website, but the data protection rules don't allow us to list any doctors as LDN prescribers without their permission. So, the physicians who are on the website now—and there are quite a few—are only the tip of the iceberg because the majority (and there are thousands worldwide who prescribe LDN) haven't given their permission. As a result, I have volunteers who are helping me contact these doctors to ask, "Would you like to be listed on the website?" We also have a volunteer who produces our videos, one who does the sound for the radio show, and another who helps get advertisers, sponsors and exhibitors for our conferences. We have a lady who sends out faxes, and another who updates the website.

We have memberships as well because we don't get any formal funding. Nobody takes a salary—everyone is a volunteer, me included. Everything we do—the website, bulk emails, our forum, conferences, recordings—costs money. So, member contributions help pay for what we offer the public.

We need more volunteers because, honestly, I am getting weary. We also need donations. I hope people who are reading this will go to our website and sign up to volunteer[62] and/or make a financial donation to support our efforts.[63]

Lastly, I'm working with Dr. Jarred Younger, who conducted the LDN fibromyalgia trials at Stanford, to raise money for a full-scale clinical trial for MS. We want it to be a very robust trial tracking many patients over a long period of time. It should be a double-blind, placebo-controlled trial that nobody can pull apart. You can't get around it. That is the establishment; that is the way things work. You can do your own thing in the background like we are doing now. But you're not going to reach the main bulk of doctors unless LDN is written about in their books and medical journals. That will only happen through clinical trials. I don't yet know how I'm going to raise the money, but I'm committed to doing it.

As you can see, I wear many hats, and I'm working hard to make LDN a household name.

There is no doubt in my mind that Linda's efforts have, indeed, turned LDN into an "almost-household name." I hope that reading her story here will encourage more people to join her—along with the many other LDN advocates and heroes—to help in the important goal of raising LDN awareness.

SECTION III:

THE STORIES

INTRODUCTION

Introduction to the LDN Stories

In this section, you will hear from 14 people—seven from the US, and seven from Europe—who have been helped by LDN for ten conditions as far ranging as Crohn's disease, rheumatoid arthritis, chronic fatigue syndrome and Parkinson's disease. Some of our contributors suffered from more than one autoimmune disease, both or all of which were helped by LDN. It would have been impossible to include success stories about all the conditions LDN might help, since there are over 200.[64]

As with all autoimmune diseases, conventionally trained doctors try to shut the immune system down with medications, on the theory that the immune system is overly active. This is contrary to Dr. Bihari's approach. He believed that shutting down the immune system is the wrong way to treat autoimmune diseases. A better way, he posited, was to "orchestrate" or "modulate" this very sensitive system, causing it to work better. This is what LDN does.

With most autoimmune diseases, conventional doctors most often start with steroids, which are very hard on the system, and which shouldn't be taken long-term. After steroids, doctors go to other drugs, many of which are toxic and side-effect laden. Some, like Gilenya for multiple sclerosis (MS), can cause a deadly brain infection, progressive multifocal leukoencephalopathy (PML). Others—biologics such as Humera, Stalera, Remicade, and

Enbrel—are used for several autoimmune diseases, and can also have horrific side effects, including cancers such as lymphomas. If these drugs don't work, doctors often turn to chemotherapy drugs such as methotrexate.

The patients profiled in this section all found LDN through their own research.

The first set of stories are from eight patients who were helped by LDN for one condition. The second set features six patients who were helped for more than one condition.

In some cases, such as chronic fatigue syndrome (CFS), fibromyalgia, Crohn's disease, and rheumatoid arthritis, we have contributions from more than one patient.

In addition to these 14 contributions, three of the LDN Heroes featured in Section II also told their own LDN stories: Frank Melhus described how his personal success using LDN to treat yet another condition—optic neuritis—led him to create his highly successful documentary for Norwegian television. Fritz Bell described how LDN helped his wife Polly, when the conventional MS drugs available at the time only made her worse. And Linda Elsegood described how her successful use of LDN for her own MS led her to create her charity organization dedicated to educating the public about it.

As you will see from reading the following contributions, in most cases, these patients were prescribed toxic drugs before finding LDN. In most cases, after finding LDN, they were able to stop taking their conventional medications, or at least, to reduce their dosages.

Now, to the patient contributions!

Contributors with One Disease

CHAPTER 7

Lad Jelen, Crohn's Disease

I'm not sure when I first met Lad Jelen. But I believe it was through Facebook, since he was active in the LDN groups there. It became obvious that Lad was eager to tell the world about his success with LDN, and I was happy to help him tell it. Lad's journey is especially compelling. It took him 53 years from his first symptoms—and 49 years since his Crohn's diagnosis—to finally find LDN. Lad wanted to do his part so that other people wouldn't have to suffer the way he did before finding LDN.

Lad and I first communicated by email in October of 2013, and spoke on the phone a month later, when he told me his story. Tragically, he died in March of 2014 from a probable heart attack. I called his wife Peggy to offer my condolences, and she told me Lad had been very proud to have his LDN story included in this book.

So here, with Peggy's help, is Lad's story. Despite the tragedy of losing Lad, his story is inspiring.

∽

I was born in 1941 and grew up on a farm in Medina, Ohio. Living on a farm, we ate a lot of natural food and drank unpasteurized—or "raw" milk, as they call it these days.

In 1956, when I was 15, I started getting abdominal cramps and spent a lot of time bent over in pain. My father, being a farmer, didn't understand; he thought I was slacking. They put me in Medina Hospital for a week, but the people there could not make a definitive diagnosis. I had a lot of discomfort going through school.

I moved to Cleveland, Ohio, and started college at Case Tech. I had a lot of difficulties with stomach problems there, too, as well as problems with a fistula.[65]

In 1959, I married my first wife, and we had an apartment in Cleveland. I was still experiencing pain, so we called a physicians' referral line, and they sent a doctor to make a house call. The cardiologist gave me something to make me more comfortable and told me to come into his office the next day. He was the first person to properly diagnose my disease which, at the time, was called regional enteritis. It later became known as Crohn's disease. This was 1960. He treated me first with prednisone and then, with ACTH gel (ACTHAR gel). He gave me the ACTHAR gel because the prednisone was causing my adrenal glands to shut down. So, periodically I would take a shot of ACTHAR gel, which was supposed to give my kidneys a kick so they wouldn't go to sleep permanently. I went on like this for years.

Then I got worse, and I had a series of abdominal resection surgeries, including in 1962, 1965, 1968, 1972, 1975 (I almost died with that one), and in 1980. Then from 1980 to 2000, I went into a "quiet phase," and didn't have any symptoms for 20 years. I am told this sometimes happens with Crohn's disease—that you can go into spontaneous remission, only to have it pop back up again years later. And sure enough, in 2000, my symptoms returned with a vengeance.

I had to have another surgery in 2000 because I was bleeding. As a matter of fact, except for 1972, when I had an obstruction, my chief symptom was always bleeding. My most recent surgery was in 2012. With that one, I had an intestinal infection, but the analysis conducted by the local hospital's lab didn't pick up the kind of infection. I went to the University Hospital of Cleveland and saw Dr. Jeffry Katz, who handles tough cases of Crohn's and other digestive diseases. He diagnosed the correct infection and started me on the right antibiotic. The problem was that, by the time Dr. Katz correctly diagnosed me, I had developed an internal fistula.

All the time when I was having resections, they were taking out parts of my digestive tract. With each of these surgeries, the primary reason was either bleeding or an obstruction. At first, with my surgeries in the 1960s, they told me, "We took out extra bowel because we wanted to make sure we got all of it." Today, when they do surgery for Crohn's, they take out only the least amount necessary.

Altogether they took out about half of my digestive tract, leaving me with symptoms of "short bowel syndrome," meaning frequent infections and diarrhea. It seemed like I was taking Imodium all the time to slow the diarrhea down. It didn't work. "Short bowel syndrome" is a mechanical thing: When you have a shortened bowel, you pick up more infections because your immune system is not working properly.

Throughout this time, they prescribed many different drugs, but none of them worked. The prednisone and the ACTH gel only suppressed the symptoms. They also tried Pentasa, which is very expensive; it didn't work either. Then they tried Azulfidine and Asacol. Nothing worked.

Finally, from around 2000 until 2008, a doctor started me on Remicade infusions. I was on this medication for a total of eight years; it worked for about six. Every eight weeks, I'd get an infusion, but its effects began to wear off after seven weeks, then after six weeks. It was problematic because I'd go six weeks with good control, and then for two weeks before the next infusion I'd be in agony. I asked my doctor to give me the infusions sooner, but he said no, that was the protocol: only once every eight weeks.

Life was difficult. Every time I'd go someplace new, the first thing I'd do would be to find the bathroom, so I could hurry there quickly when I needed to go. It was a very limited life. There were many things I couldn't do that I had enjoyed before—like camping—because I might have difficulty with my digestion or not be able to find a bathroom. I got along, though. My pain was often there in some form or another, but at least it wasn't constant.

All this time, I held two jobs. In 2000 I lost my main job: quality engineer for a manufacturing company. They had a cutback, and I was laid off. But I still had my secondary job, working at a drugstore.

I had another surgery in 2000. Afterwards, I tried to go back to work at the store, but my Crohn's was so bad I could no longer handle a full shift. I told them I had to quit and filed for Social Security Disability benefits. It took the better part of two years for me to get approved, but I finally qualified.

After that, I was still having lots of problems, so finally, I started researching Crohn's disease on the Internet. I thought that maybe I could qualify for some trial of a new drug. I saw that Penn State University was conducting a clinical trial of a drug called Low Dose Naltrexone (LDN). I looked it up on the Internet and saw that many people were experiencing a lot of success with it. I called Penn State and asked them if they were still recruiting. They said there were two trials in progress, one for adults and one for children, and that both were double-blind studies. So, there was no guarantee that I'd get the medication. I might be getting the placebo.

In January 2009, I drove 720 miles round trip to Penn State, and they put me in the trial, handed me a bottle of capsules and told me to start taking them. I did. I was in so much pain that after one week I called them and told them it wasn't working. They told me to try to make a go of it until my next appointment in a month. I tried for another week, then called them back and said, "It still isn't working." I told them that if I couldn't get something that worked I would be dropping out of the trial. They got nervous.

When I went in the next time, I repeated what I had said on the phone: "This stuff isn't working, and if you don't give me something that works, I'm going to have to drop out of this trial." I told them

I couldn't keep traveling 720 miles round trip to feel this bad. They took mercy on me and broke the seal—it was a sealed trial.[66] They came back and said, "You might have been on the placebo."

I said, "I'm sure I was!" It turns out I was right. Originally, they had planned to give me the placebo for three months and then the real drug for another three. They gave me another bottle, which turned out to be LDN, and sent me home.

Within a week I started feeling much better. It was amazing how quickly I turned the corner.

After being on LDN for six months, I had my Crohn's Disease Activity Index (CDAI) tested. My CDAI—which gauges the activity of the disease—was 450 when I started the trial. By the end, it was 150. They said that 150 was the indication that I was in remission.

I told them I'd heard that people were having problems getting prescriptions for Low Dose Naltrexone and asked if they could help me with that. Dr. Jill Smith, the doctor running the trial, gave me a year's prescription. I did fine for that year. Then I tried to get another prescription from another doctor, and I had a lot of trouble. This doctor was associated with the Cleveland Clinic, one of the top medical centers in the country. He told me that according to his contract with the clinic, he was not allowed to prescribe anything off label. He could prescribe Cimzia, Remicade, and all those other drugs. But, according to the rules of his contract, he could not write me a prescription for Low Dose Naltrexone.

I had to find an independent doctor who would write me a prescription. But even doctors who were not at Cleveland Clinic wouldn't prescribe LDN for me. It took me three more tries before I finally found a doctor who was willing to listen to me, and who also had experience with Crohn's disease. He just asked me: "What do you need?" I told him I needed a prescription for Low Dose Naltrexone, as well as a few other prescriptions and he said,

"Done!" He gave me a year's worth of prescriptions, including one for LDN. I sent it off to Skip's Pharmacy in Boca Raton, Florida, and Skip promptly came through with what I needed.

I want to stress that when I went to each of the doctors who turned me down for LDN, I told each of them about the clinical trial. I told them that the trial drug had worked and put me into remission. I brought in the information I got off the Internet about LDN and how it works. They all refused to write me a prescription for LDN. And still, they would have been willing to give me prescriptions for the other Crohn's drugs—many of which I'd been on before, and all of which hadn't worked.

I think the problem *isn't* that Low Dose Naltrexone is off label. I think the real problem is that as soon as doctors hear the word "naltrexone," they think "drug abuse." There's a stigma attached to naltrexone.

I'm doing fine now. The problem is that because I have so much of my bowel missing, I have short bowel syndrome. But other than that, I'm doing okay. I'm more or less normal now. I can lead a normal life. I am very happy.

I take a few other medications, including metronidazole (Flagyl) for the short bowel syndrome. I understand that a lot of Crohn's people take this drug since short bowel syndrome causes us to develop infections easily. I also take blood pressure pills for my high blood pressure. I have stage 3 kidney disease, and I have a nephrologist following that. And osteoarthritis. I have a lot of "old people's diseases." But my Crohn's is under control.

My primary care doctor was very understanding about the pain I was having before I went on LDN. Even though she wouldn't write me a prescription for LDN, she did write me prescriptions for narcotic painkillers. I managed with that and Tylenol before I got the LDN prescription. Now I don't need painkillers at all.

I have a friend at church who has breast cancer. They took off one breast, then the other. Then it went to her bones. She's now on Low Dose Naltrexone for her cancer, and it's in remission.

A problem with all this is that you can only do a clinical trial for one drug, one disease. You may know that a drug is useful for something else, but no one will discuss it because they're making so much money on other drugs. I read an article about Low Dose Naltrexone that called it the "most misunderstood drug of all time."

I am really "out there," spreading the word about LDN. My main avenue is Facebook, especially the groups for IBD[67] and Crohn's. I don't measure my success by people's response to me. I just want them to know LDN works for me, and it may work for them. The difference LDN has made in my life is amazing, and I want to see if it makes a big difference in other people's lives, too.

[Author's Note: Dr. Jill Smith was willing to clarify the part of Lad's contribution that was unclear: his claim that the directors of the trial had "broken the seal." She recommended keeping Lad's version of his story "as is"—including his belief that the study directors had "broken the seal," and offered to add her "official take" on the situation. Here is what she said:

> We didn't exactly take mercy on Lad. Although we did care about him, we really were following the protocol. There was nothing we did for him that broke the protocol or, in his words, "broke the seal," although that was his interpretation. According to the protocol it says, "During the first three months of the study, if a subject has a flare-up in Crohn's symptoms or an increase of at least 100 points on the CDAI score, the subject will be given the option of being rescued with steroids and dropped from the study or switched to the active drug if on placebo." So, we didn't unblind the study. The pharmacy knew what Lad was getting—i.e., the naltrexone or the placebo—but we didn't know. When he came in

and was having a flare up, and his CDAI went up by a hundred points, he was eligible to either drop out of the study and have us give him steroids or stay in the trial and get the drug being studied. If he had originally been getting LDN and was not doing well and said, "I want to continue on the study," the pharmacy would have re-dispensed naltrexone to him, and he would have continued doing poorly. But, since he was getting the placebo and wasn't doing well, he was absolutely eligible to get the LDN. And as he stated, he started feeling much better almost immediately!]

I hope that Lad's story will be read by many people who have been recently diagnosed with Crohn's disease. Finding LDN sooner could help people with Crohn's stop the progression of the disease. With early intervention, Crohn's disease patients could potentially avoid the kind of debilitating surgeries Lad underwent. If Lad's story helps even one Crohn's patient find relief with LDN, I know he would have been happy.

CHAPTER 8

Maija Haavisto, Finland, Chronic Fatigue Syndrome/ Myalgic Encephalomyelitis

I am not exactly sure how I first learned about Finnish writer, Maija Haavisto. It seems that I have always known about her work concerning LDN. But when I delved further, I learned that she is an expert on so much more. Maija is, in fact, one of the foremost researchers and writers about treatments for chronic fatigue syndrome. Having a difficult-to-diagnose illness turned Maija into a tenacious medical detective—first for herself, and then for countless others. I am honored that she has agreed to tell her story for this book.

In her words:

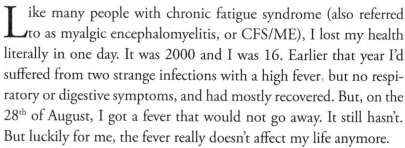

Like many people with chronic fatigue syndrome (also referred to as myalgic encephalomyelitis, or CFS/ME), I lost my health literally in one day. It was 2000 and I was 16. Earlier that year I'd suffered from two strange infections with a high fever, but no respiratory or digestive symptoms, and had mostly recovered. But, on the 28th of August, I got a fever that would not go away. It still hasn't. But luckily for me, the fever really doesn't affect my life anymore.

The fatigue wasn't initially very bad, but it started getting worse almost from the beginning and steadily worsened further over time. The name "chronic fatigue syndrome" is misleading, since some people don't suffer from "fatigue" at all. I did, though—along with a host of other symptoms that appeared insidiously. Among the first were palpitations, muscle weakness, swollen lymph nodes and migraines. Some of my friends were worried that I had leukemia, while others assured me it was probably just psychosomatic. My parents believed the latter.

I was keen to believe the psychosomatic explanation myself. I was having a very stressful time at home, and my mother frequently threatened to throw me out. I wasn't a problem kid, but I was never good enough to meet her expectations. In November 2000, she finally kicked me out. I was lucky to find a job as a freelance journalist, writing for a computer magazine, so I was able to support myself.

I was elated. I figured that if my condition was caused by the stressful home situation—and surely it must be—it would soon get better and my fever would go down. But I just kept getting worse, and a host of new symptoms appeared, including absence seizures,[68] insomnia, nausea, vision disturbances, dizziness, neuropathic pain, chronic urticaria (hives), chest pain, breathing problems and constant bacterial infections. Both my memory and concentration were also affected, and I couldn't work very much—just barely enough to support myself. I'd leave off words when speaking and writing. All these symptoms were very frightening to me.

"Chronic fever" is an elusive term, difficult to explain. Medical textbooks with a chapter about "fever of unknown origin" usually list only cancer, infections like tuberculosis and some autoimmune diseases as potential causes—but not CFS/ME, even though it's among the most common causes for prolonged fever. Some people told me they thought I didn't really have a fever, just "elevated body temperature." I'm not sure exactly what they meant by this, but I think some of them thought my temperature wasn't high enough to be considered a real fever. Others believed that an elevated body temperature was normal for me. But it sure felt like a fever. I'd get horrible chills and would pile myself with clothes and blankets. I'd often add towels on top of them, to keep myself warm, even in the summer. When the fever started going down, I'd sweat profusely. But it never went away.

In early 2002 I first heard of fibromyalgia. Out of curiosity, I started Googling it, even though I knew I couldn't have it since I didn't suffer from pain. Fibromyalgia websites led me to CFS/ME, which sounded just like what I had, complete with a sudden onset after a viral infection. Not many illnesses start like that. Mine did.

It might have been a relief since I was finally pretty sure I knew what was wrong with me. But this wasn't good news since CFS/ME wasn't considered curable, and many people ended up in wheelchairs or even being tube fed. A few also lost their cognitive function, to the point where they weren't able to understand speech or recognize family members. Some even died. It was clear to me that my illness was progressive. Would I end up in a wheelchair? I had always been more of a reader and writer than an athlete, so I was even more terrified of losing my cognitive abilities.

There was another huge problem for me in that CFS/ME was virtually unknown in my home country of Finland, despite the fact that myalgic encephalomyelitis had been identified as a disease in 1969 by the World Health Organization (WHO) after multiple epidemics occurred throughout the world. By the 1950s there were reports of CFS/ME epidemics in the US, the UK, Australia, Switzerland, Denmark, Greece, and Iceland. And, according to many authorities, it was up to five times more common than MS. Still, it was virtually unknown in Finland.

I went to see several doctors, but none of them had heard of it. They told me my fever would go away if I stopped thinking about it. One GP ran an ECG, which the computer analysis found very troubling. It showed inverted T waves, suggestive of past myocardial infarction. I was 18. But my doctor told me it was nothing to worry about—that I should just exercise more.

Years later I found out he had tentatively diagnosed me with viral myocarditis, an infection of the heart muscle, for which the only "treatment" is to *avoid exertion*. I have no idea why he gave me such bad advice. Luckily, I was aware that in CFS/ME, exercise can be extremely dangerous—so I didn't heed his advice.

For a few years, I gave up on doctors. I was sure I'd just be wasting what little money, time, and energy I had. I was still deteriorating. I continued researching treatments on my own, but the brain fog got much worse. I couldn't really read books anymore, just magazines. On my worst days, I'd browse through ad catalogs, desperately bored and pretending I was reading something. Luckily ginkgo biloba, which I began taking on my own, helped alleviate some of my cognitive problems if I took it religiously three times a day. If I missed one dose, I would notice.

But my cognitive fatigability was still severe. Writing made me feel like my brain was fried. I couldn't think at all. Mental exertion was actually worse for me than physical exertion, though physical exhaustion could make me feel extremely ill for a week.

I couldn't find any relief for my other symptoms, either. Would it ever be possible to find something to stall the progression of my illness? I began to doubt it. It just didn't seem likely that an herb or vitamin would do that, or that I could find a doctor willing to prescribe something for me.

In late 2005 I got an email from the wife of a Finnish CFS/ME patient. Her husband had been diagnosed at the infectious disease clinic of Helsinki University Hospital. And he had actually gotten treatment there! It sounded too good to be true in a country where you couldn't find a single website devoted to or even mentioning this illness, except for one page of information from a university hospital in northern Finland. But, information about CFS/ME wasn't in any magazine or newspaper, or on any health website. There were no organizations...no numbers to call.

I followed her advice and went to see the doctor in charge of the infectious disease clinic privately, meaning I had to pay for the visit. Most health care in Finland is on the public sector, which is cheap or free, but waiting times can be massive, and you also need a referral for specialists. Privately I was able to see this specialist without a referral. He agreed that I probably had CFS/ME and wrote me a referral for the clinic, which was on the public sector, so I didn't have to pay anything for the large number of tests he had me undergo. One time they took 25 tubes of blood. I also had ultrasounds of my heart and stomach and a chest X-ray. The clinic finally gave me the diagnosis of chronic fatigue syndrome.

I'm not sure exactly where I first heard about LDN. It might have been from a book about CFS/ME treatments I read back in 2004 or 2005, or even before that on the Internet. When I read about the positive experiences of people with MS who took LDN, I was intrigued, since the way MS progresses seemed quite similar to my progressive CFS/ME. I asked for it at the clinic, but they refused to prescribe it for me.

The doctors offered me prednisone, a steroid. It is not commonly used in CFS/ME, and a study done in the early 1990s found it to be no better than a placebo. But for some reason, they used it for CFS/ME then and still do, even though it very rarely helps anyone and is actually much more dangerous than LDN.

As a strange coincidence, in the past, my dad had given me a few prednisone pills to try for my chronic urticaria, and it had made me feel much better, almost healthy. So, I knew prednisone would help me, even though it helps very few people with CFS/ME. I also strongly suspected that its benefit might be short-lived and that the side effects might be terrible. The doctors didn't actually tell me about the side effects, but I was aware of the risks. I knew it was a bad idea to take it.

Nonetheless, I started prednisone on the last day of 2005, and as far as steroids go, it was surprisingly kind to me. I got hardly any side effects, except for a little weight gain, particularly the rounded "moon face" typical of corticosteroids, and some occasional joint pain. I felt very good. My fatigue was much relieved, and the fever didn't really bother me. I had my life back, but I was almost certain it wouldn't last. It didn't.

In late spring of 2006, I told the doctors that prednisone's efficacy was waning, and they instructed me how to wean myself off slowly. It was a nightmarish ordeal that lasted for eight months and caused symptoms like low appetite, low blood sugar, stomach pain, nausea, and severe joint pain. With each dose reduction, I'd spend three weeks almost bedridden, then a week slightly better. Then it would be time to reduce the dose again, which meant a new cycle of feeling horrible for three weeks.

The computer magazine I worked for went bust in the spring of 2006. I applied for sick leave and then disability, but because of my CFS/ME diagnosis, the Finnish public insurance provider said I was perfectly healthy and denied my application. You see, they didn't accept CFS/ME as an actual illness, even if you were completely bedridden. Although I wasn't bedridden, I wasn't well enough to go to court to protest their decision. So, I only qualified for minimum income support. And because of my young age, the welfare office sent me forms to fill out about my "drug use" and "criminal history." It was humiliating.

Shortly before I started the prednisone withdrawal, I built the first Finnish website for CFS/ME, which included a forum.[69] I decided I'd compile a booklet of medications used in CFS/ME treatment that I could put on the website as a PDF. Through my research, I'd read about many types of treatments. Some of them weren't available in Finland, but many were, from antihistamines to antivirals and Alzheimer's drugs. I included all of them—along with LDN—in the PDF.

The project grew so large, with well over 100 medications, that I decided I would self-publish it in 2007 as a book,[70] the original Finnish version of what was to become *Reviving the Broken Marionette: Treatments for CFS/ME and Fibromyalgia.*[71] The English version was published in 2008. It was ironic that I knew about so many different drugs like LDN that were shown to help people with CFS/ME, but the doctors at the infectious disease clinic wouldn't prescribe any of them for me. They had a short and rigid list of drugs they would prescribe, most of which had no evidence to back them up and some, like prednisone, which actually had negative evidence.

My physical condition continued its rapid decline. Very abruptly I began to lose my ability to walk. I remember standing at the door of a small supermarket and wondering if I could make it through. It looked like I'd soon be in a wheelchair, provided I was even able to get one with my "diagnosis *non grata.*" I loved cooking, but even preparing the simplest dish, or stirring soup, could land me in bed for the rest of the day. Filling out a complaint form about yet another day of sick leave laid me flat for 18 hours, made worse by the fact that I could barely tolerate light. The official board that handles public insurance disputes dismissed all my complaints. In the meantime, my cognitive problems continued to worsen, making it harder to keep writing my book and maintain my website.

In early 2007 I heard of a promising sleep doctor on the online forum I had started, which is still in existence today. He was considering trying infliximab, a biological TNF alpha blocker, on another CFS/ME patient. I didn't want an immunosuppressant, which infliximab was, but I knew I needed an open-minded doctor, which he seemed to be. So, I made an appointment to see Dr. Olli Polo.

We clicked right away. I told him about my CFS/ME book and about LDN. He had never heard of LDN, but it made sense to him since he was in the process of reviewing a student's PhD dissertation relating to endorphins and the immune system. Remember, LDN modulates the immune system and raises endorphin levels.

I walked off with that precious prescription I thought I'd never get. I tried not to get my hopes up too high since I knew that nothing works for everyone. At that time, LDN hadn't been used that much for patients with CFS/ME, so no one knew how often it did work. In the past few years LDN has become more and more of a "standard" drug for CFS/ME and fibromyalgia, used all over the Western world. There is even a Facebook group for patients with CFS and Fibromyalgia.[72]

I took my first dose on the evening of March 5, 2007. I had mild sleep disturbances, a slight tremor in my legs, and I woke up at 6:00 a.m., feeling very hungry. But, despite the sleep deprivation, I was already feeling better. I could take notes by hand without feeling like dying afterward. By the second night, the minor side effects no longer bothered me.

That weekend I went dancing.

Things were definitely improving for me! The hallmark of CFS/ME, severe post-exertional malaise (PEM), was no longer a part of my life. I could do whatever I wanted without worrying about repercussions lasting for days. Maybe I didn't even fit the diagnostic criteria anymore since I no longer had PEM. My muscle weakness was much less severe. The fever hardly bothered me anymore, either. Even though I was and still am running a fever all the time, it's mostly asymptomatic, *in that I no longer get chills or feel feverish*. My lymph nodes are no longer swollen and achy. The chronic urticaria has disappeared. My exercise-induced asthma, which I had experienced ever since I was a child, has lessened, too, as have my other breathing troubles. And I no longer suffer from constant bacterial infections.

LDN didn't help all my symptoms, though. MS patients often experience improvement in urinary frequency, but I didn't. My cognitive dysfunction was only somewhat relieved, but luckily my doctor agreed to prescribe piracetam and nimodipine—"nootropics," or "cognition-enhancing drugs"—for me, which lifted the fog and allowed me to write productively again and to speak and write without dropping words.

Life was good again. Really good. Thanks to LDN, I could walk 10 kilometers on a good day. This was hard for me to believe; before LDN, I had struggled to walk just a few meters.

In 2009, I got a contract with a Finnish academic publisher to revise and update the Finnish version of *Reviving the Broken Marionette*. It was published in 2010. Dr. Polo wrote the foreword, focusing on LDN. He had prescribed it for another patient the same week he wrote my script and was soon using it as a first-line treatment for both CFS/ME and fibromyalgia. Patients were flocking to his office for LDN prescriptions!

Soon Dr. Polo was prescribing it for approximately 1,000 other patients with CFS/ME, as well as for a few with fibromyalgia and other autoimmune conditions. Unfortunately, in 2017, he got into trouble with the Finnish medical authorities,[73] who accused him of prescribing too much of one "experimental medicine." It is unclear whether the authorities were referring to LDN, since one of the representatives put in writing that the loss of his license had nothing to do with LDN. But the upshot is that he lost his license and cannot prescribe LDN until the situation is cleared up.

In 2010 I traveled to Glasgow, Scotland, and Birmingham, England to speak at two LDN conferences about my own and other Finnish patients' experiences. In August I got married, and in September of that year, I moved to Amsterdam with my husband, a long-time dream for us. I signed the contract for my debut novel—also about CFS/ME—titled *Marian ilmestykset*[74] (*Maria's Book of Revelations*), as well as for a new medical book about little-known and poorly understood chronic illnesses and their treatments. This second book is titled *Hankala Potilas Vai Hankala Sairaus*[75] in Finnish, which translates to *Difficult Patient* or *Difficult Illness*. (The title does not translate into English very well.) I also adapted my novel into a play, which was in production in 2014 in Finland for three weeks, and we are currently seeking funding for a movie based on this play. We have a director who has his own production company and is eager to direct it. But, in Finland, governmental organizations basically fund all feature films, because even hit movies have a limited audience because of the country's small population. We are still attempting to secure funding.

Dream after dream was coming true. I could hardly believe it.

A few years ago, I appeared on a major Finnish TV talk show discussing CFS/ME along with my doctor and another CFS/ME patient, who had also been helped by LDN. Unfortunately, they cut out the parts where I explained the benefits of LDN in MS and other conditions, but its usefulness in CFS/ME came through loud and clear.

I want to be clear that LDN doesn't help every single health problem on the planet. Sadly, I've amassed some illnesses that LDN cannot treat, like hypopituitarism, and more recently, gastroparesis, which means food moves too slowly through my GI tract. But still, after being on LDN for over a decade, I've accomplished and experienced quite a lot in my life for someone with a serious illness. I've had seven novels published, along with three medical books, two other non-fiction books, a poetry collection, and a children's book. I've also written about medical topics for some major Finnish magazines and given quite a few interviews. [Author's Note: There is an up-to-date list of Maija's publications online at http://www.fiikus.net.]

Over the years I've tried dozens of other treatments to improve my overall functioning. I've benefited from several, including the previously mentioned nimodipine and piracetam, as well as pyridostigmine, testosterone, supplemental oxygen, and many herbs and supplements. But other treatments that have helped reduce my fatigue or muscle weakness or have enabled me to work more, invariably stop working for me. Sometimes they have helped for just a few days, sometimes for a few years, but usually, they help for only one to two months. No doctor has been able to figure out why they stop working. Treatments that benefit my sleep, migraines or cognitive function do retain their efficacy.

But out of all the supplements, medications and other types of treatments, the only one that still helps my fatigue, and still helps me walk after all these years, is LDN. I can still walk several kilometers a day, but not ten, as was often the case right after I started taking LDN.

When people ask me: "Is LDN still working for you?" my answer is always: "Definitely!"

∽

Each of this book's contributors has gone out of his or her way to spread the word about LDN. For years, Maija has used her extraordinary writing skills to educate the public about it. I am grateful to her for agreeing to tell her story for this book.

CHAPTER 9

John O'Connell, Hashimoto's Thyroiditis

I learned about John O'Connell from Dr. John Sullivan, a Mechanicsburg, Pennsylvania physician who was an LDN-prescribing doctor for many years. Dr. Sullivan put me in touch with John, who referred me to his YouTube videos.[76][77] *I watched them and knew that his story needed to be shared.*

John, who now resides in upstate New York, lived near Annapolis, Maryland at the time of our first interview. He retired in 2005 at the age of 52 after a long career as an analyst with the Department of Defense, tracking government contractors to make sure they did not overcharge for extra parts or labor.

Here, in John's own words, is the story of his years of illness before he finally found LDN in early 2012, as well as the dramatic results he has experienced.

∼

In 1993, when I was 40, I was diagnosed with hypothyroidism, an underactive thyroid. This diagnosis was not a surprise because, when I was born, my mother suffered a serious form of hyperthyroidism, an overactive thyroid. My father later told me that the doctor said that because of my mother's hyperthyroidism, I was likely to develop the opposite condition, hypothyroidism, at some point in my life.

Upon diagnosis, I was prescribed levothyroxine, a synthetic form of thyroid medication used to treat hypothyroid. At the time, it didn't seem like a big deal to me. It was just another medication I had to take as I moved into middle age. Everything went along fine for the rest of the 1990s with very few changes in my condition, except that it was becoming tough for me to keep my weight down. As a result, I was always on a diet of some sort: Jenny Craig, Weight Watchers—I must have tried them all.

But suddenly, in September of 2002, I noticed a significant change. At my father's 80th birthday party in Florida, I experienced the first instance of something I call "a nerve weakness attack" in my feet that made it difficult for me to walk for long periods or distances. Looking back, I see that this was probably the first symptom of my Hashimoto's thyroiditis, the autoimmune disease of the thyroid that is a common cause of hypothyroidism. But I was not diagnosed with Hashimoto's for another seven years.

During the seven years from 2002 to 2009, I had six or seven flare-ups of nerve weakness of varying severity, mainly affecting my feet and hands. Each flare-up lasted from one to three weeks before gradually subsiding. The neurologists I consulted couldn't figure it out. They tested me for both diabetes and multiple sclerosis, but the tests always came back negative. They determined that these attacks were "idiopathic," meaning "unknown cause." I thought that maybe I had a vitamin deficiency, or something else equally insignificant.

However, some of these nerve attacks were so severe that I was unable to stand or walk for long periods of time. I had diminished dexterity in my fingers, sometimes making it difficult to handle keys, button a shirt, or even operate my smartphone. During three of these severe episodes, I decided to go to the emergency room for help. But with each attack, they referred me back to my neurologist who performed more tests. I went to three different neurologists between 2005 and 2009, but each of them said that the tests only showed I suffered from "idiopathic neuropathy."

Between 2002 and 2009, another marker for my yet-to-be-diagnosed Hashimoto's disease developed gradually: the loss of almost all the hair from my legs and arms. My eyebrows also shortened at the ends. Eventually, my eyebrows covered only about 75 percent of the area above my lids.

In 2009, I asked to see a thyroid specialist and was referred to Dr. T, a board-certified endocrinologist. She did a diagnostic panel, including the thyroid peroxidase antibody (TPOAb) test, which detected my autoimmune Hashimoto's thyroiditis. Dr. T gave me a basic informational pamphlet describing the disorder, but told me there was no cure, and instructed me to keep taking levothyroxine. I didn't pay much attention to the pamphlet or grasp the seriousness of the diagnosis. She made the disease sound standard and utterly routine.

From late 2010 into 2012, further problems developed. In particular, my legs below the knees became weaker, and I experienced more swelling in my feet and legs. I continued to see Dr. T until she left the area. At that point, since Dr. T hadn't been doing anything other than prescribing levothyroxine, I didn't see a need to consult another endocrinologist and went back to my primary care doctor.

Life was becoming increasingly difficult. The weakness in my legs was making it hard for me to stand or walk for any length of time. My legs were like sticks, weak, and almost unable to support my weight. I was unable to do my usual, everyday tasks, such as going to the store to get groceries. I started two types of diuretic medications, metolazone, and furosemide, for the swelling. But that was it.

Although I had the leg weakness and swelling issue for some time after my diagnosis, I still didn't associate them with my disease. The symptoms were staring me in the face, but I didn't recognize them.

Then, in the summer of 2011, I began seeing Dr. C, a chiropractor near my home in Maryland. I thought that some stenosis that I had developed in my lower lumbar spine might be making my legs weak. But after several months of chiropractic treatment, there was no improvement. In fact, I seemed to be getting worse. Dr. C authorized an MRI of my lumbar spine and arranged for the results to be reviewed by Dr. N, a neurosurgeon.

I saw Dr. N in January 2012. He gave me a physical exam and reviewed my MRI results. By this time, my legs had become so weak that I bought an $800 electric cart that I kept in the car to use at grocery and department stores. It was terrifying. I was convinced that, at the age of 58, I was becoming so disabled that I was headed for a wheelchair-bound life. Even more frightening, I lived alone and feared I'd eventually end up in an assisted-living facility.

Dr. N didn't note anything in my MRI that could be causing my significant leg weakness. However, he did note the swelling of my legs and feet, as well as the hairlessness of my legs, as symptoms that might be related to my complaints.

The doctors weren't coming up with any new information to help me. Following this examination, I decided I'd better start researching my Hashimoto's thyroiditis because I became convinced that these frightening symptoms I'd been developing were probably related.

The best site I found detailing Hashimoto's symptoms was FreeMD.com. Here, for the first time, I saw a detailed list of symptoms—many that I had experienced myself since 2002. In particular, I learned that bilateral leg and foot swelling, leg weakness and loss of body hair are all common Hashimoto's symptoms.

Further online research showed that Hashimoto's is *progressive*, and as with most autoimmune diseases, there is no known cure. This was depressing. But I finally had an explanation for what was wrong with me. I realized I'd made a big mistake in not researching from the start.

In January 2012, I began researching what, if any, treatment options were available for Hashimoto's. YouTube turned out to be a valuable resource. You have to be cautious because there is a great deal of false and misleading information on YouTube. But it's certainly a good starting point. At least, it was for me. Purely by luck, I came across Joseph Wouk's three informational videos about Low Dose Naltrexone (LDN). Joseph—the son of author Herman Wouk (*Winds of War*, *The Caine Mutiny*)—had a severe case of multiple sclerosis. Through his research, he stumbled on LDN and found it to be an effective treatment for his rapidly declining health. (He later published a book, *Google LDN*,[78] in which he maintains that LDN is a viable medical treatment for people afflicted by all sorts of autoimmune disorders, not just MS.)

I began hungrily researching to learn everything I could about LDN. I read two books cover to cover: *Up the Creek with a Paddle*[79] by Mary Anne Boyle Bradley, and *The Promise of Low Dose Naltrexone Therapy*[80] by Elaine A. Moore and Samantha Wilkinson. I was most impressed with Ms. Bradley's book, in which she documented how LDN slowed the progression of her husband Noel's multiple sclerosis. But the most important lesson I learned from these two books was that, if LDN was to work for me, time was of the essence.

I also discovered that even if LDN was not a cure for my disease, if it worked for me, LDN could achieve two goals:

1. Stop or slow the progression of my disease
2. Slow, halt, or reverse some recent symptoms

Since my inability to walk and stand for any length of time was such a dramatic, recent symptom, it was clear that I had to give

LDN a try very soon or resign myself to the rest of my life in a wheelchair. This was not an acceptable option!

In early February of 2012, I decided to try LDN. At the time, I was seeing only my primary care physician, Dr. P, who was responsible for all my medications. I approached him with some basic research materials and asked about trying LDN. Unfortunately, he ignored my research and told me he wouldn't consider prescribing LDN for me. I sensed that, since LDN is not mainstream medicine, Dr. P had no interest in learning about it. I was disappointed, but frankly, I wasn't surprised.

I had learned from my research that, because of the lack of interest in LDN by the big pharmaceutical companies—there is no profit potential in LDN—there hasn't been substantive research or support for LDN from the medical community. As a result, the conventional physicians who know about it consider it to be an alternative therapy and, in fact, most physicians don't know about it at all. I don't know Dr. P's reasons, but he wasn't interested.

However, *The Promise of Low Dose Naltrexone Therapy* included the names of physicians knowledgeable about LDN. One was Dr. John S. Sullivan in Mechanicsburg, Pennsylvania. I made an appointment to see him. After reviewing my medical records and performing a physical, Dr. Sullivan prescribed LDN for the treatment of my Hashimoto's thyroiditis. It was March of 2012.

I didn't experience any immediate reaction to the medication. However, within three months of taking LDN at the recommended dose of 4.5 mg, my primary leg weakness started gradually to go away. When I was experiencing the symptoms of Hashimoto's and could hardly walk, I still tried to exercise at my local gym, where I had been a member for a few years. But, over time I'd been able to do less and less and had to modify my exercise routine to avoid leg workouts. But after I started taking LDN, I was able to resume almost daily hour-long workouts without any problem at all. It was great to be able to do my usual exercises using the elliptical machines and treadmill! It seemed like a miracle!

Most of my other symptoms—leg swelling, foot neuropathy, and difficulty losing weight—improved too, but to a lesser extent. These are, however, longer-standing symptoms that dated back to 2005, and some symptoms—for instance, the nerve problems—dated back to 2002. I knew from my research that I probably couldn't expect much help for the oldest symptoms. Since starting LDN, however, I haven't had any recurrences or flare-ups of nerve attacks involving weakness of my feet, hands, or fingers. No trips to the local ER, either. That is the absolute truth. I'm feeling so much better!

About a month before starting LDN, I went to see a podiatrist because I had a tumor in my foot. It disappeared after I started taking LDN. I believe LDN got rid of it because there is no other explanation for its disappearance. My podiatrist was stunned; you should have seen his face.

I am sure that without LDN these past five years, I would now need a wheelchair and would be in an assisted-living facility or nursing home. I have had no illness at all during that time. Not even one cold.

And another thing I can tell you that shows the power of LDN: In 2010, before I started taking LDN, I had a colonoscopy, and it was bad, showing ten polyps. I was classified as being at high risk and in need of further follow-ups. In 2014, after two years on LDN, a follow-up colonoscopy revealed no significant irregularities, and I was reclassified as low risk, and would not need another colonoscopy for ten years. By then, I'll probably be too old to need one anyway. Just further confirmation to me that LDN fixes the immune system and works.

I'm very grateful to authors Joseph Wouk, Mary Bradley, Elaine Moore, and Samantha Wilkinson for helping me to discover the benefits of LDN therapy when I did. I believe that LDN is as close to a "miracle drug" as you can get. There is nothing else out there that I know of that is as effective against such a wide variety of autoimmune diseases and works so cheaply—and with an absolute minimum of side effects. I've been on LDN for six years now—long enough to judge its effectiveness. However, you must be the judge if LDN is right for you. Ultimately, it's your health and your choice.

In October 2013, John attended an LDN conference in Schaumburg, Illinois—a conference I also attended. It was gratifying to meet him in person and to see how well he was doing—walking on his own without even a cane. And there was no trace of the electric cart! John is active on Facebook, especially in the group, "Beating Thyroid Disease with LDN," answering questions from other people with thyroid disease and telling the other members about his success with LDN. I often "meet" him there!

Also, the disappearance of John's foot tumor was likely the result of the LDN, which successfully treats many people with tumors and cancer. Dr. Bihari reported many instances of LDN's bringing about remissions in cancer patients.[81] [82]

CHAPTER 10

May-Britt Hansen, Netherlands, Hailey-Hailey Disease

While all the other contributions to this book are by people with diseases with easily recognizable names—Crohn's, Parkinson's, rheumatoid arthritis, fibromyalgia, etc.—May-Britt Hansen's chapter is the exception.

Like several of my other contributors, I first met May-Britt on Facebook, and took notice of her when she shared the news in October 2017 that LDN had actually made it into the mainstream medical press (JAMA[83] Dermatology) as being an effective treatment for the very rare skin disease, Hailey-Hailey disease, or HHD. It was a condition I had never heard of.

The fact that LDN had made it into JAMA was big news!

May-Britt told me how LDN had helped her with her HHD and, in passing, with the pain associated with her fibromyalgia and osteoarthritis, as well. We decided that she would tell her story, but she would concentrate on her Hailey-Hailey disease since she felt it was her most devastating, challenging and life-changing condition. I asked her to share her contribution for this book.

Here is May-Britt in her own words.

My LDN journey began in November 2012. I suffer from a rare genetic skin disorder called Hailey-Hailey disease (HHD). It is a painful blistering skin disease in which the skin layers don't adhere like they should, so the skin literally falls apart like a brick wall collapsing. This causes blistering which later turns into painful weeping open wounds, which often become infected. The wounds are often compared to burn wounds. HHD is usually an inherited disease, but no one in my family is known to have it.

I went through several misdiagnoses before getting the correct diagnosis of HHD in 2011. I had suffered a massive outbreak after a nasty flu, which probably caused my immune system to be compromised. It started with spots and blisters on my back, which turned into very painful sores. My doctor diagnosed me with shingles. The pain was so excruciating that it kept me from sleeping. My doctor gave me an antidepressant called amitriptyline—frequently prescribed for shingles patients—to ease the nerve pain.

Soon my sores started to spread to my chest and upper stomach, as well as under my breasts. Pretty much my entire upper body was covered, and the blisters turned into oozing open wounds and cracks in my skin. There was a strange smell coming from the wounds. I was at my wit's end and went back to see the doctor. She was also shocked and concluded that this was not looking like shingles; maybe it was herpes simplex. She told me to continue taking the amitriptyline, as well as an antibiotic, and to come back in two weeks.

Things got worse instead of improving, so I was given five rounds of antibiotics. But I didn't improve, so finally my doctor decided that, since these medications were not helping, we needed to find out what kind of infection I had. So, she did a swab test. The results came back showing I had a staphylococcus infection, not herpes simplex.

Because I was feeling so miserable and was so exhausted from the pain, I was referred to a dermatologist. But the dermatologist didn't know what it was either, so he did a biopsy to see if it was some form of skin cancer. It was extremely stressful emotionally—

almost unbearable—to have a biopsy performed on open wounds. I dreaded it.

But thankfully, the biopsy results didn't show any signs of cancer. Instead, I learned I had Hailey-Hailey disease. I had never heard of it, and my dermatologist knew nothing about it, either, other than what he read. Even worse, what he read made him very uncomfortable.

He told me I had an incurable disease and that there was little he could do for me, but that I should avoid friction, sunbathing, and sweating. Easier said than done when the temperature was 34° Celsius (93° Fahrenheit)! I was sent home with a prescription for a corticosteroid cream.

Five months had gone by since I had experienced my first symptoms. I was extremely frustrated; I felt helpless and totally worn out emotionally. My family tried to be supportive, but no one could understand what I was going through—especially since my clothes were hiding my symptoms. I applied the cream two to three times a day, but it didn't seem to do much. My clothes often stuck to my skin and I had to soak them off in the shower. If I didn't do that, they would rip my skin off.

It became a vicious cycle of new sores, skin accidentally ripping apart, deep cracks, weeping wounds, dry crusts, itching, and pain. I gave up hope of ever healing again. Simple things like going grocery shopping and driving became almost impossible because I always felt like my skin was being ripped apart. Bending and stretching were nearly impossible, too. Taking care of my wounds took up a huge amount of my time. My days of being able to shower and apply body lotion were over. My new ritual was soaking my shirts, carefully showering, and then applying corticosteroid cream and bandages, which also had to be soaked off.

I stopped the amitriptyline since it didn't help with the pain and instead took painkillers that didn't help either. Sleeping was impossible. I was only able to sleep for an hour at the time.

Miraculously, after nearly ten months, my wounds stopped spreading and started to dry out. I was relieved. But I was also scared that my symptoms would come back.

By now, I had been searching online for information about HHD, but there was very little out there. After a few clear weeks, I let my guard down and became used to a symptom-free life once again. Life was wonderful. Unfortunately, as I had feared, my clear period lasted a little less than four months. When the blisters appeared again, I felt lost and knew what was coming. I hadn't known that the first time.

Thinking back, I had had milder symptoms over the years, but didn't know it was HHD: small scratches, blisters and sores under my breasts and on my behind in the summertime, caused by sweating and friction.

Soon I had full blown HHD again. This time I just accepted that there was little to nothing to be done except the usual creams and bandages. The only difference was that I didn't have a secondary infection this time. I got a prescription for tramadol for the pain. It felt heavenly to go from a pain level of 10 to a 7. If you are in constant pain, you don't aim to be pain-free. You learn to settle for less pain.

At this point, I just wanted to stay in bed and at the worst, not to wake up anymore. But I couldn't do that because I had a household to run and people who depended on me. My mother, who has since died, was my rock and an amazing support.

After a few months, I made another appointment with the dermatologist and again was told there was little to be done. I got a cream called silver sulfadiazine that was soothing and antimicrobial and was told to use it, along with the corticosteroid cream, and to cover my wounds with a bandage or Mepilex plasters. Again, I accepted that there was nothing to be done. It was very unusual for me to be so passive, but I guess it shows what a disease can do to a person emotionally.

I was so tired of everything and felt so disgusting with all these wounds on my body. I couldn't do anything without planning. It affected my social life in so many ways. For instance, because of the pain I was experiencing, I could no longer go out with friends as often; and because of the fatigue, tasks that were once easy to do became difficult. I had to give up sports, which I had enjoyed before, because of the sweating and friction. I could never leave the house spontaneously; I always had to take precautions—for instance, choosing clothes that would not cause me too much pain.

In September 2012, I began searching on Facebook to see if I could find anything about HHD. I was surprised to see there was a support group. I can't describe how it felt to be accepted into a group made up of fellow sufferers. I cried because of all the compassion and understanding after all the time I had spent alone with this disease. HHD patients often suffer alone unless other family members show signs of the disease. People feel ashamed to have a body that is covered with sores and the purple scarring the sores often leave behind.

It was in this group that I first heard about LDN. Two people were taking it and having good results. I was desperate and willing to try anything. I decided I wanted to try LDN. I researched online to understand what LDN was and how it worked. I joined two LDN Facebook groups, the LDN Research Trust group, and "Got Endorphins? LDN." I made another dermatologist appointment and told him about LDN. He had never heard of it and said he'd have to discuss it with his superiors. I had told him I would get LDN one way or the other, with or without him. My fighting spirit was back!

The hospital did another biopsy which again confirmed that I had HHD. After two weeks I got approval to start LDN. After conferring with his superiors, the dermatologist told me to take a 50 mg tablet and break it into four pieces and start with 12.5 mg. But I explained that I needed a 1.5 mg tablet. (I don't react well to taking capsules.) After much discussion, he finally wrote a prescription for that dose but told me not to have any expectations. He took pictures of my wounds and said he would call me in two weeks to see how things were going.

I started LDN at the end of November 2012 and noticed a change within two weeks. My sores weren't spreading, and they slowly began to dry. When the dermatologist heard this, he wanted to see me after two more weeks on LDN.

After one month on LDN, I experienced a 50 percent improvement and was very excited to see my dermatologist. The look on his face was priceless when he saw my wounds and compared them with the photos he had. He was very excited and admitted he hadn't had any expectations when I started LDN and only went along with prescribing it for me because I was so determined and had told him I would find a way to get it anyway, without him. He had felt very uncomfortable with that idea.

We agreed that I should continue LDN and scheduled an appointment for one month.

By the end of January 2013—after only two months on LDN—I was totally clear. The dermatologist was very excited, and we agreed to make a new appointment in another three months unless I had a new outbreak. After three months I was still clear and only needed to see him every six months. Sometimes a small blister would try to pop up, but it usually went away within a few days.

Around that same time, another surprising thing happened: I noticed that pain from two other conditions I'd suffered with since my late twenties and had gotten progressively worse over the years—fibromyalgia and osteoarthritis—had lessened significantly after LDN. Surprisingly, I had never read anything about LDN's positive effects on pain.

Miraculously, my HHD remained stable. After one year, by the beginning of 2014, I was still clear and only needed to see my dermatologist once a year. In 2016, he dismissed me as a patient and told me to call in the event of an outbreak.

I am happy to report that there has been no need to call him. I have learned so much since 2012 and know a lot more than when I was first diagnosed with Hailey-Hailey disease.

I wanted to do something for my fellow sufferers, so I became even more involved in the online HHD community. When the original HHD Facebook support groups became inactive, we started a new one, The Hailey-Hailey Disease Worldwide Support Network—at https://www.facebook.com/groups/HHDWSN—where we encourage each other and share our knowledge—both general and relating to LDN—with those who are new to this disease.

In October 2017, two small case studies on LDN for HHD were published—one in *JAMA Dermatology*, conducted at Emory University in Atlanta (https://www.ncbi.nlm.nih.gov/pubmed/28768313); and the other in the *British Journal of Dermatology* (https://www.ncbi.nlm.nih.gov/pubmed/28991360). This is encouraging news. Because of the Emory study, dermatologists throughout the world are prescribing LDN for their HHD patients. So, people with HHD now have better access to LDN.

There is officially no standard treatment for HHD, and LDN is certainly a powerful alternative to the more toxic and often ineffective medications that are usually prescribed: antibiotics, prednisone, acitretin, corticosteroid creams—and even methotrexate, a chemotherapy drug.

I don't take any other medicines for my HHD, and my skin has been clear since January 2013, except for a small blister now and then which I can hardly call an outbreak. I do take precautions, though: I wear clothes made of soft fabrics, prevent friction and sweating, and shower twice a day. I also avoid stress as much as possible, eat a healthy diet, and limit my sugar intake.

I never take for granted that things will stay as they are at the moment; I realize my situation could change overnight. But for me, LDN has been life-changing.

Since my diagnosis in 2012, many more people with HHD are now taking LDN. Most have good results: fewer and less frequent outbreaks; also, fewer infections with the outbreaks.

My wish for the HHD community is that everyone who wants to try LDN will get the chance to do so.

Thank you for letting me share my HHD/LDN story.

In a recent conversation with May-Britt, she told me that she currently takes 3 mg LDN and feels that it is the best dose for her. She took 4.5 mg for a short while, but it did not work as well for her as 3 mg does; it gave her headaches. She changed to 3 mg in mid-2014. For May-Britt, less is more. She is also happy to report that she has been able to lower the doses of the pain medications she used to take for her fibromyalgia and osteoarthritis. While she used to have to take the NSAID naproxen almost every day, she now only needs it a few times a month. So LDN has helped her in more ways than she ever hoped for.

CHAPTER 11

Andrea Schwung, Germany, Multiple Sclerosis

Like so many of the contributors to this book, I first met Andrea Schwung on Facebook, where she is an administrator of the German LDN group, LDN Low-dose Naltrexon (Deutschland)—https://www.facebook.com/groups/315938001858805/. When I decided I wanted to include contributions from LDN users around the world, I posted a request in her group for submissions. Andrea was quick to respond—and even supplied her story in English, which was a great help to me.

This is Andrea's story.

∽

I consider myself lucky that my doctors in Germany discovered quite early on that I had a form of multiple sclerosis (MS). However, the process to find a treatment that helped me—and that I was comfortable with—took more time.

This is my story.

In December 2004, I was being treated for back problems, for which I had already had surgery. But now, I was having symptoms I was quite sure were not back related: I couldn't wiggle my toes, and I had trouble climbing stairs. My symptoms moved up my body to the point where lifting my arm to blow-dry my hair was more difficult than it had been before.

So, I went to the hospital in December. I had just turned 42.

I had an MRI. The doctors were puzzled by what they saw. The MRI showed multiple lesions in my brain; one—the most active lesion—was as big as a golf ball. This explained why my walking and lifting my arm were impaired to the point where I resembled a stroke patient. My lumbar puncture confirmed that it was MS. But all the doctors who saw me—and my scans—were confused about the kind of MS it was. They still are. But they all agree that it is some form of MS, no matter which terms they use to describe it.

After receiving my first infusion of high dose steroids, I was able to wiggle my toes and, a bit later, to walk around, with difficulty.

The doctors urged me to start Interferon therapy as soon as possible. I did this for two and a half years but had another MS episode six month later. In large part, though, my symptoms went away with steroids.

While I was still on the Interferon therapy, I continued to suffer from a slight dropping or stamping of my right foot when I walked. I had experienced this during my first MS episode in December of 2004. I was able to walk for 20 minutes, but then the weakness would return, and I would need to rest.

I was not content with this form of therapy—Interferon and steroids—or with living this way.

So, after two and a half years of once-weekly Interferon therapy, I stopped it. The side effects—high fever and flu-like symptoms—had not been pleasant, and anyway, I wanted to see what would happen if I went off the medication.

But six months later I had another episode: I had trouble seeing and was prescribed steroids again. Even though I was still resistant to going back to "mainstream" medical treatment, I took steroids. And again, they did the trick. I was fine—for a while.

I had another episode not long afterward. This time my speech was affected. Again, steroids helped.

My doctor urged me to start Interferon therapy again. He was afraid that the steroids would lose their magic and that, every time

I would have another episode, I would become immune to their effects. I opted not to take the Interferon therapy.

In the spring of 2008, I discovered the website, LDNinfo.org, and became a member of the Low Dose Naltrexone Yahoo Group, where I communicated with many people and learned of their successes taking LDN. I thought that this medication seemed almost too good to be true. But after doing my own research, I became very hopeful about trying LDN.

I had known this doctor—the same one who had recommended Interferon in December—for four years, and he trusts me. I printed out the informational packet from the LDN website and gave it to him. He had never heard of LDN but agreed to write me a prescription. At first, he prescribed a 50 mg naltrexone tablet, called Nemexin in Germany, and I made my own LDN, using information I found on the Internet. I started with 4.5 mg in liquid form. After a few weeks, I decided that it would be easier just to take a pill, so I ordered 4.5 mg capsules from Skip's Pharmacy in Florida. Thank goodness Skip was able to ship LDN internationally!

I started taking LDN in the summer of 2008. For nine years, I didn't have any MS episodes. However, just recently, this past September, after nine years of no symptoms, I had another episode, with minor problems with my fine motor skills. I detected the problem very quickly, was put on steroids again, and my symptoms went away. I changed my LDN dose from 4.5 mg to 3 mg and am doing my best to avoid gluten and cut down on meat!

My symptoms have totally disappeared once again.

From the time I first started using LDN in 2008, I became a member of the online LDN community, at first, to learn more about this inexpensive, off-label medication. Then, I became more active, first with the Yahoo LDN group. Then I started my own German LDN Yahoo group. In 2013, a woman named Isabella Bella convinced me that Facebook was a better venue than Yahoo.

She started the German Facebook group and made me an administrator. I am now the most active administrator of the group, which is quite lively. Through it, I help promote, educate, inform and—most importantly—make people aware of this wonderful off-label medicine for the many forms of multiple sclerosis, as well as for other diseases that LDN has been proven to help. I want to add that the German LDN Yahoo group still exists, and I sometimes participate in it. But since I believe Facebook is a much better venue for online conversation, I mostly concentrate on Facebook.

One of the members of the group is Stefan Heider, a compounding pharmacist in Germany. His pharmacy, City Apotheke, makes capsules for most of the members of our group, and he offers a discount to our members. His site is located at: http://www.cityapotheke-goettingen.de/apotheke.

I still go for yearly checkups to my same doctor, who conducts a variety of tests and has kept a 12-year record, since my original diagnosis.

He is amazed—even astounded—by what LDN has done for me, and if any other patient wants it, he has no problem prescribing it.

I am happier, healthier, and still, to this day, very lucky.

[Author's Note: Andrea is multicultural. Born in Germany near Düsseldorf, she now lives in Madrid, Spain. Over the years, she has lived in New York, Moscow, Shanghai, and Tokyo. So, many of the visits to hospitals and doctors described here took place in several countries.]

When Andrea hears about the problems other people are having with MS, she considers herself to be very lucky. What a wonderful story—a 13-year-plus saga—of how LDN has helped her to stay happy and healthy. And her German LDN Facebook group continues to grow every day.

CHAPTER 12

Emiliano Marchi, Italy, Multiple Sclerosis

Without a doubt, Emiliano Marchi is the person who has done the most to spread the word about LDN in Italy. He is the creator of the Italian LDN website (http://www.ldnitalia.org), and administrator of the Italian LDN Facebook group, "Gruppo LDN Italia" https://www.facebook.com/groups/189026731227. I asked him to tell his personal story of how LDN has helped him with his MS—and how he went on to help others in Italy to learn about LDN.

He told me he is honored to be a part of this book. I am honored to have him.

Emiliano shares his story.

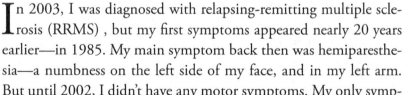

In 2003, I was diagnosed with relapsing-remitting multiple sclerosis (RRMS), but my first symptoms appeared nearly 20 years earlier—in 1985. My main symptom back then was hemiparesthesia—a numbness on the left side of my face, and in my left arm. But until 2002, I didn't have any motor symptoms. My only symptoms were lack of sensitivity to touch, double vision, and difficulty emptying my bladder.

No one ever mentioned multiple sclerosis (MS) to me.

In September 2002, on a business trip in Argentina, I started to have problems with my left leg. Intermittently, it was stiff and awkward. When that happened, I had trouble walking.

When I returned to Italy, I was very worried that I had MS. (I had studied medicine for two years and knew the symptoms.) So,

I consulted a neurologist. He told me it was not MS, but for some reason, he ordered a tomography of my brain, without contrast. It turned out negative, as I knew it would. I knew I needed an MRI, so I found another neurologist, who ordered one. It uncovered several small lesions. Afterward, he hospitalized me; they performed several studies, including an EEG and a lumbar puncture. Although these tests were inconclusive, all my symptoms progressed over the next six months to such an extent that my neurologist told me I had RRMS.

At first, I did just what my neurologist suggested: In the summer of 2003, he started me on the Interferon, Betaseron—three injections a week. The side effects were terrible: headaches, flu-like symptoms, fever, exhaustion, and muscle weakness in my legs. All activity was impossible for me because of the fatigue. After less than one year, I could no longer tolerate the side effects.

When I told the neurologist how awful my side effects were, he prescribed two cycles of the immune-suppressing chemotherapy drug, mitoxantrone (brand name Novantrone).

The side effects of this drug were even worse than those of Betaseron. And even so, my disease progressed. But the worst part was that one of the possible long-term side effects of mitoxantrone is cancer, especially leukemia and melanoma. Eleven years later, in April 2016, I had surgery in my right arm for a melanoma. The dermatologist said it was because of the mitoxantrone I had been given eleven years earlier.

After experiencing the horrible side effects and complications from the two conventional drugs I had been prescribed, I decided to search the Internet for an alternative therapy. In 2007, I found the US website, LDNinfo.org, which contained a link to the Yahoo LDN forum. I wrote to Dr. David Gluck, creator of the website, and also the forum's administrator, and asked him for information about LDN, which he sent me. I decided I wanted to try it.

I asked people in the group how I could get LDN in Italy. One member told me about making my own LDN with distilled water from a 50 mg tablet. I told the group that in Italy there was a product called Antaxone, which is naltrexone hydrochloride liquid, which I could get from any pharmacy in 10 ml bottles; each bottle is equivalent to one 50 mg tablet. Several members agreed that this would be a good option.

I needed to get a prescription for Antaxone. I went first to my neurologist, who did not support my decision to take LDN because it is not a standard therapy for MS. So, I changed to a neurologist who was knowledgeable about it and gave me a prescription for Antaxone. I started at 1.5 mg and gradually increased it until I reached 4 mg. That dose proved to be too high; it caused stiffness and spasticity, so I lowered it to 3 mg. Then, sadly, after three years of prescribing Antaxone for me, my neurologist died. Although my current neurologist agrees with my taking LDN, he says he can't prescribe it because it is off-label for MS. So, I found a homeopathic doctor who writes my prescriptions.

For the past six years, I have been taking 3 mg capsules, which my homeopathic doctor prescribes for me. The first supply I got was from Skip's Pharmacy in the US, and I used Skip's for a year. But having any medication sent from a country outside Europe is a problem for customs here in Italy. It involves paying extra money and filling out lots of paperwork. Fortunately, now there are compounding pharmacies in Italy that compound LDN, so starting two or three years ago, I began using an Italian pharmacy. Skip taught me how to make the LDN capsules—which fillers to use, etc.—and I explained it to my pharmacist.

There are now seven compounding pharmacies that make LDN in Italy, and the number is growing. We list them on our website. http://www.ldnitalia.org/come%20ottenere%20naltrexone.htm

Thanks to LDN, my life has changed completely for the better since 2007. I no longer have any MS symptoms or any major problems with fatigue. After my first week on LDN, I felt so much better: no more tiredness or weakness; and no more problems with walking, bladder, or balance. In fact, I have no limitations of any kind. I am a different person—and everyone I come in contact with who knew me before remarks on the change LDN has made in me.

I am now retired and devote myself to my favorite sport: I'm a master at karate! I am separated from my wife, and my 33-year-old twin sons, Yuri and Elvis, live with me. I do all the housework, go to the grocery store, and do most of the cooking. I travel around Italy taking my students to competitions everywhere without problems. All this would have been impossible before LDN.

In 2008, I created the Italian LDN site, http://www.ldnitalia.org. Dr. Gluck told me he'd be honored to give me permission to use the information from his US site, http://ldninfo.org. He provides a link on his site to ours, and we provide a link to his, as well. Linda Elsegood also links to our site from hers, LDNResearchTrust.org.

I have become so enthusiastic about LDN that in November of 2009, I started the LDN Facebook group, "Gruppo LDN Italia." https://www.facebook.com/groups/189026731227

Thanks to both the Italian LDN website and Facebook group, there are now many LDN users in Italy. Also thanks to my online presence, several neurologists in Italy now trust me, and are beginning to prescribe LDN for their patients with MS; one neurologist prescribes it for other autoimmune conditions, as well. Some non-neurologists in Italy, who learned about LDN from our website, also prescribe it for their patients. I would never have believed any of this could have happened when I first learned about LDN.

In addition to karate, spreading the word about LDN is my life!

∼

Thanks to Emiliano's devotion to LDN, his Facebook group now has nearly 1,000 members, and several hundred people in Italy now take LDN for illnesses such as MS, rheumatoid arthritis, Crohn's disease, and even cancer. Emiliano receives at least 10 phone calls a week from people who want to take LDN, and just as many emails and calls from people who tell him that he has saved their lives. He always corrects them, by telling them that LDN— not he—has saved their lives!

CHAPTER 13

Lexie Lindstrom, Parkinson's Disease

I first learned about Lexie Lindstrom in 2013 from journalist Larry Fuchsberg, who answered a press release that was sent out about my book, Honest Medicine, *by my publicist, Cathy Lewis. The release was about how LDN helps people with autoimmune diseases at a fraction of the cost of most drugs doctors prescribe. Larry wrote that he wanted a copy of my book, adding that he had recently been diagnosed with Parkinson's disease (PD), and was about to start taking LDN.*

I was surprised and curious since, although I had heard that LDN had helped many people with PD, I didn't know of any actual cases.

I asked Larry how he learned about LDN for PD. He said he had heard a woman named Lexie Lindstrom speak about her success with LDN at the Third Parkinson's Recovery Summit in Santa Fe a few months earlier. He told me to Google the conference and Lexie's name, which I did. Before I knew it, I was listening to an interview with her,[84] and was determined to hear her story firsthand. I tracked her down.

Since then, Lexie and I have become fast friends. Here is her story.

∽

I was diagnosed with Parkinson's disease in October 2008, when I was 60 years old. But looking back, my symptoms started 20 years earlier, when I totally lost my sense of smell. I was later to learn that many patients lose their ability to smell several years before being diagnosed with Parkinson's. But, since I'd had a 30-year professional career in the cosmetic and fragrance industry, I chalked this up to what I referred to as "olfactory system burnout" and didn't think much about it.

All my life, I'd been healthy, active and relatively fit, and almost never got sick. I rarely, if ever, got a cold and only had the flu once in my adult life. Although I hardly ever got sick, I was no stranger to stress and anxiety, which I was later to learn is a huge factor in Parkinson's disease.

Stress began for me at an early age when my parents divorced. And it continued to overwhelm me throughout my childhood. I worried about everything and everybody: my mom, my dad, my two brothers. I became the family worrier early on. My father died at 71, and my two beloved younger brothers died suddenly and unexpectedly five years apart when they were 44 and 51. Their deaths devastated me.

Then, in 1988, when I was 40, a major trauma turned my entire world upside down. I was on the receiving end of a divorce I didn't see coming. I was crushed and dumbfounded. What I thought was my perfect life ended abruptly. At the time I was working full time for a prestigious cosmetics company in Training and Education. I thanked God that I had a career I loved so that I could distract myself from my new reality. But my divorce put me into a tailspin. I was hanging on by a string emotionally.

Soon after my divorce, I started having new and unusual symptoms that I attributed to stress: severe anxiety along with equally severe, chronic insomnia. Another new symptom was irritable bowel syndrome (IBS) with constipation, which started getting worse and worse. I also had this horrible, embarrassing urinary incontinence. Again, I thought all these symptoms were triggered by the stress from my divorce and never considered that it might be something more serious.

I dealt with each symptom separately, going to a different doctor for each one. A psychiatrist prescribed an antidepressant for my anxiety, and a sleep specialist prescribed sleep medication for my insomnia. My gastroenterologist told me to eat more fiber for my IBS and constipation. These treatments and suggestions helped somewhat. But, my urinary incontinence, which was so bad that I had to wear pads, was hard to understand because, from what I read, the condition is more common in women who have had children. I saw a urologist who diagnosed me with "neurogenic bladder spasms." I asked him what could have caused this condition in a person who had never had children. He said my bladder spasms were most likely "idiopathic," meaning "of unknown cause."

I didn't like being told that my symptoms were idiopathic. They had to be caused by *something*! I asked him which medical conditions could cause bladder spasms. He said it might either be multiple sclerosis or Parkinson's disease.

This was the first time I'd ever heard either disease mentioned as a possible cause of my symptoms. I knew that both conditions were very serious, so I was alarmed when the doctor mentioned them as possibilities. The urologist asked me if I had any symptoms of Parkinson's disease, but didn't tell me what those symptoms were. To me, Parkinson's meant "only tremors," so I said, "No, I don't think so." And he didn't question me about it any further. He referred me to a neurologist who specialized in MS for an MRI. The MRI showed that I didn't have MS. That was such a relief. Thinking back, I'm not sure why we didn't pursue the possibility of Parkinson's disease at this time. But we didn't.

The urologist offered to give me medication for my bladder spasms, but I'd read about this side-effect-laden drug and had seen ads for it on TV. I refused the medicine and decided to continue wearing pads, hoping my incontinence would improve.

Eight years after my divorce, I married a man who was wonderfully compassionate and supportive. I also made a major career change, moving into the medical arena in cosmetics sales, calling on plastic surgeons, dermatologists, and spas. During all this time I continued to live with my symptoms, with no clue that my real problem was anything other than stress.

The stress in my life continued to build. In 2003, shortly after my second brother's passing, my mom, who was also my best friend, was diagnosed with Alzheimer's disease, which she suffered with for nine heartbreaking years before passing away in 2012. In addition, I had career stress caused by my perfectionist personality and my determination to be a high achiever. I was driven to succeed and worked very hard regardless of the toll it took on my health and wellbeing. Stress had really morphed into every area of my life, but I just thought that was normal for me. Little did I know at the time that this almost constant stress, along with my perfectionist nature and drive to succeed, were the earmarks of what is known as a classic "Parkinson's disease personality."

In 2008, my life took a dramatic turn. In October, I was sitting in the bathtub, and my right big toe was tremoring. I said to my husband, "Look at my toe; it's shaking." It was weird. We were both perplexed. We lived on a farm and, shortly after that, I was walking from the barn to the farmhouse and noticed that my right foot wasn't picking up. It was dragging. I was tripping, and the only way I can describe the feeling is that it was like my brain wasn't telling my foot to lift up high enough when I was walking. I tripped and fell several times. I had to be very careful about going upstairs because I was falling on the stairs. At around the same time, I saw myself in the reflection of a large window and noticed my right arm was not swinging naturally like my left arm when I was walking. I thought that was odd. But it was my tripping and my right foot dragging that caused me the most concern. This definitely was not normal.

I thought this was a brain issue—a neurological issue of some kind. I made an appointment with a neurologist in the town where I lived and got in to see him as soon as I could. He watched me walk and noticed that my right arm didn't swing. I told him I had been tripping, that my foot wasn't lifting up and that my right toe had been tremoring. I also told him about all the other non-motor symptoms I'd been having. He had me perform a few tests and asked me some questions. Then he matter-of-factly said: "You have Parkinson's disease." I was stunned and devastated. I had heard the word Parkinson's from the urologist a few years before, but I thought we had ruled it out as a diagnosis. I asked him if he was sure, and he said, "Based on all your symptoms, I would say yes."

I wanted more information and asked him if he felt there would be a cure for Parkinson's in my lifetime. He shook his head and said "no." At this point, I didn't really trust him entirely, probably because he was very curt with me. I was his last patient of the day, and he didn't seem to want to spend time explaining things. When I asked him if he had any information about Parkinson's disease that he could share with me, he just said, "You can look it up on the Internet. You're savvy."

I decided not to go back to him. But I did want a second opinion to find out for sure whether or not I had Parkinson's. I made an appointment with the neurology clinic at the Mayo Clinic in Scottsdale, Arizona. I thought, "This is where I'm going to get a definitive answer." The neurologist at Mayo went through all the same tests and asked me lots of questions. I was in her office for about an hour and a half. In the end, she said, "It sounds like you have Parkinson's disease."

I asked if any special tests would prove definitively that I had Parkinson's. She said there was one test that would give a more definitive answer and sent me over to the hospital the next day for a lengthy examination where they put electrodes all over my body to test for internal tremors. On that particular day, I wasn't tremoring noticeably. I told the neurologist who was administering the test that I didn't always tremor. He said it wouldn't matter; the test would still be able to detect internal tremors.

Sure enough, the test picked up tremors all over the right side of my body. I was finally convinced that I had Parkinson's.

Back at home, it was time for me to find a neurologist who would be my doctor. I didn't want to go back to the local neurologist, because I thought his bedside manner was terrible. And the neurologist at Mayo was too far from where I lived. I needed a doctor I liked who was closer to me. I researched and found the best movement disorder specialist (MDS) I could find in Seattle, Washington, close to where I lived and made an appointment to see her.

My new doctor was top-notch, highly regarded. In fact, she is the neurologist I still have today. I trusted the medical institution she's affiliated with since it's one of the top medical facilities in the state. I also trusted the physicians there. On my first official appointment, she confirmed my diagnosis and did some physical and mental testing.

I reluctantly agreed that the time was right for me to start taking one of the Parkinson's disease medications since my condition was affecting my work so badly. My neurologist said I had a couple of choices. First, there was the "gold standard" medication for Parkinson's: Sinemet (Carbidopa-Levodopa). She said it could control the majority of my symptoms quite well, and that with it I would be able to live a fairly normal life for the next five years, or maybe longer. The most startling part that she didn't mention, but that I soon found out through my research, was that, at the time, this "gold standard" drug was 45 years old and would do nothing to stop the disease progression! It would only treat the symptoms. I found this very upsetting.

Maybe that was why the neurologist I'd consulted with at the Mayo Clinic in November 2008 had warned me, "Whatever you do, don't let anybody start you on Sinemet." She'd told me that there were newer drugs called "agonists," and that I should start with one of them. Her words were ringing in my ears now. I shook my head and told my new neurologist I didn't want to start on Sinemet. She looked at me and said, "Oh no, another Sinemet phobic!" She was right: I was a Sinemet phobic!

All the while, I kept thinking, "This is good news? I have five-plus years!?" I was mortified. I was a young, active 60-year-old woman. What I had just learned meant that for the next five years, or maybe longer, I would have "good symptom control." But what would happen to me after that? Sinemet seemed to me like a 45-year-old Band-Aid for a disease with no cure. I knew right away that this drug was not for me. Not then anyway, and hopefully, never. I waited to hear about my next option.

As my doctor at Mayo had suggested, my next option was an "agonist." My new doctor recommended Requip. Unfortunately, I experienced some very unusual and troubling side effects that are now known to affect a significant number of Requip patients. First, it caused me to become a shopaholic—an addiction that could have ruined my marriage. I don't think I had ever been inside a Goodwill store before, but suddenly I had this obsession with shopping there. I spent hours at our local Goodwill and bought lots of household items and clothes I didn't need. It was a nightmare. My doctor smiled when I told her, and we agreed that it was good that at least I wasn't shopping at Nordstrom's!

My husband would call, and I'd lie, telling him I was shopping for groceries. At the time, I just couldn't figure out why I'd developed such a shopping addiction. I didn't realize that the Requip was causing it. I'm surprised it's still on the market since it has many disturbing side effects for so many people who take it.

But Requip had another much more dangerous side effect for me. I began falling asleep while driving. This happened four times in rush-hour traffic on the freeway before my doctor agreed that Requip wasn't a good option for me. I must have had an angel on my shoulder because I never hit anybody, and nobody ever hit me. But my doctor finally said, "This drug is going to kill you," and put me on Sinemet.

I slowly titrated off Requip while starting Sinemet. Even though I'd been warned about it, and was so dead set against taking it, Sinemet actually turned out to be an okay drug for me. I got pretty good symptom control. But I now knew that I was truly on my own. There was no way I wanted to be on Sinemet for five years and then have to take higher and higher doses. If I was ever going to get well and do it without side-effect-laden drugs, I knew I'd have to find my own way out of this abyss.

In 2009, I started researching on the Internet in earnest. I became a "research fanatic." I soon realized that traditional Western medicine would not hold any answers for me. I started joining Parkinson's disease forums where I listened to people talk about how they were handling their disease and their symptoms. I had certainly experienced my share of scary and disturbing symptoms, so I had empathy for what these people were saying. But still, in my heart, I could not accept that disease progression and drugs would always be my fate. I could not wrap my head around having this disease forever, even though I was as sick as everyone else on the forum and—like them—was in "PD survival mode," taking medications each day and trying my best to control my symptoms and lead a somewhat normal life.

After a couple of months on these forums, communicating with people from all over the world, I began to develop friendships. We all spoke about the doses of the different PD meds we were taking, what worked best, what didn't, whether exercise was helpful, and if so, how much. Meditation and yoga were mentioned, but it was just the general stuff I guess people talk about for a "no hope" disease. We were all in the same boat, going up the same "creek without a paddle." It was good to have others I could commiserate with, but I was still looking for that glimmer of hope. My poor husband became so frustrated with me as I spent hours past our bedtime logged onto these forums, listening and posting. I had to know if there was anything promising out there.

Finally! Enter Low Dose Naltrexone!

One day, a woman named Destiny Ellen came onto the forum. She was talking about her father, who had been a professional wrestler and had PD for many years. She and her mother were devoting their lives to helping him. She said that a drug called Low Dose Naltrexone had "saved his life." Thanks to this drug, which he'd been taking for several years now, her father was having a reversal of some of his PD symptoms, and his disease didn't seem to be progressing at all! She said she only wished she'd learned about it years earlier.

I locked onto Destiny's story! Not many people on the forum paid much attention to what she had to say, except for me and a few others who rarely posted due to the controversy over "unproven" or "unconventional" treatments for PD. Most of the others in the forum were PD "veterans" who had "heard this type of thing before." Some admitted that they had spoken to their neurologists about LDN, as Destiny called it. They would all come back with the same responses from their doctors: "It doesn't work." "It's just hype."

It confounded me that these people believed whatever their neurologists said was the only truth and that most of them had no desire to step outside the box.

I just couldn't relate. Nor could I get enough of what Destiny Ellen had to say about her dad's progress with LDN. Their incredible story had been featured in an Oregon/Washington newspaper.[85] I was impressed. The way Destiny described LDN made sense to me. She and I connected on the forum, as well as by email and phone. I looked at all the LDN websites I could find online and became fascinated! Was LDN what it appeared to be: a modern-day wonder drug of the twenty-first century? If so, how could it be that our doctors *didn't even know about it?*

Destiny said I'd have to get a prescription from my doctor. Right away, I talked to my neurologist about LDN. She thought it was crazy. She said there were no clinical studies showing LDN's success for Parkinson's disease. I told her that a lot of people with MS were having fabulous results with LDN and that there were some LDN studies to confirm it. But she responded that MS was a lot different from Parkinson's and refused to write me a prescription.

At my next two appointments, I brought in lots of information I'd copied off the Internet, but she wasn't interested in looking at it.

Finally, at my next appointment, I began to cry. I said, "I have a disease that has no cure, and I'm not the kind of person who can live with a no-hope disease." I added, "I found a drug that appears to be very safe and that a lot of people are taking, and I want you to give me a prescription for it." I told her that if she didn't give me a prescription, I'd go to another doctor, but that I'd much rather partner with her. She looked at me for a few moments and finally said, "I won't write a prescription right away, but I promise to look into it and get back to you. I want to make sure LDN is really safe before I agree to prescribe it."

She called the manufacturer of Azilect, which I had recently started taking, in addition to Sinemet. (I was still titrating off Requip.) She asked the research department if it would be safe to take Low Dose Naltrexone with Azilect. They assured her that there wouldn't be a problem. I was kind of surprised that the research department at Azilect knew about LDN when my neurologist didn't.

I Start LDN!

The next day her assistant called me and said that she had approved a prescription for LDN. I was ecstatic. *I agreed to take it at my own risk.* I believe it's really important to tell your doctor you'll take LDN at your own risk because they're all afraid of liability. I was so excited that I was finally able to start taking LDN. Hope at last! I began with 3 mg before bedtime on October 24, 2009. The next day I had a feeling of wellbeing for the first time in a long time. And I had that feeling of wellbeing for the next two days, as well. I began to notice all-around symptom relief. I had much less anxiety and fatigue. A sense of calm came over me. My voice was getting noticeably stronger and less crackly sounding. My body was responding so quickly to LDN that it took even me by surprise!

Many of my symptoms kept getting better and better on LDN, including my severe anxiety, which literally disappeared. My PD symptoms in relation to balance, slowness of movement and dizziness also got noticeably better, and my PD fatigue was markedly improved, as well. Soon I was able to lower the dosages of my medications.

Nearly nine years later, I am taking 4.5 mg of LDN every night. My PD progression has been very slow, which impresses my neurologist. I recently had an appointment with her about my cognition, and it turned out well. How much of that is because of

LDN, we'll never know for sure. But I give LDN a huge amount of the credit.

I am still taking Carbidopa/Levodopa and am symptom-free if I stay on schedule with my meds every day. If I veer off schedule, my symptoms become more apparent: shaking, right foot dyskinesia and difficulty with balance. Still and all, I feel blessed to be doing so well. My neurologist says I am still in the upper one percent of her slowly progressing patients, and she gives me a year's prescription for LDN, which I have filled by Skip's Pharmacy.

Even with my remarkable response to LDN, my neurologist at first insisted that it was due to the "placebo effect," and now, years later, she says it is because of my "great attitude." It's so frustrating. Even my primary care physician, whom I have had for years, says the same thing. In the beginning, when I first started taking LDN, he said, "You're really having a wonderful placebo effect." I told him then, "But it's not a placebo effect; it's real," and he said, "Lexie, placebo effects can be very, very powerful."

I think the world of my doctors, but it's really troubling that they don't believe LDN is the reason for the remarkable control and even reversal of so many of my PD symptoms. I see patients in my neurologist's waiting room who are hunched over. They have Parkinson's so bad they're walking with walkers, and I think, "Why aren't you telling them about LDN?" My neurologist has responded to this question by saying: "There are no clinical trials for LDN for PD, so I can't recommend it." However, she now gives her patients a prescription if they ask for it.

My husband is thrilled by how well I'm doing on LDN. We both have a renewed hope for our future together.

I tell people about LDN whenever I can and share articles and information with them. I have been a four-time guest on a BlogTalkRadio Internet interview show. The host, Robert Rodgers, PhD, of ParkinsonsRecovery.com, tells me that the interviews with me are among the most popular. As a result of being a guest on this show, many more Parkinson's patients are now taking and benefitting from LDN. [Author's Note: Lexie has been on four shows with Dr. Rodgers. She invited me to be on two of them with her. All four are online.[86] [87] [88] [89]]

I am also influencing a handful of my friends with other autoimmune diseases to take LDN. They are having the same kind of success I have had.

However, many Parkinson's patients I communicate with online still don't believe me when I say LDN has made all the difference for me. I will never stop trying to get the word out to as many people as possible because I'm so grateful to have my life back and I believe in LDN so profoundly. I want to give others the chance to experience the amazing results I've had.

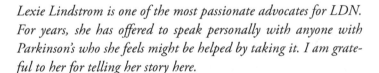

Lexie Lindstrom is one of the most passionate advocates for LDN. For years, she has offered to speak personally with anyone with Parkinson's who she feels might be helped by taking it. I am grateful to her for telling her story here.

CHAPTER 14

Maureen Mirand, Rheumatoid Arthritis

In 2013, I asked Diane Kruger, administrator of the Facebook group, "LDN for Rheumatoid Arthritis Disease," to help me find a contributor for this book who was successfully using LDN for rheumatoid arthritis (RA). Diane put out a call for contributors. Maureen Mirand answered, saying: "I was diagnosed with severe, aggressive RA in 2011. I couldn't turn my head or walk without a struggle and felt sick all the time. I could barely get off the couch and was in such pain I thought I would lose my mind. I never took methotrexate, though, even though the doctors wanted me to take it. I found the LDN website, found our support group and spoke with Skip Lenz. Finally, my doctor allowed me to try LDN, and I have been doing very well."

Here, in her own words, is Maureen's story.

∼

I'd been tired for as long as I could remember. I had many stressors in my life, including having triplets and dealing with my husband's cancer. But I was tired even as a child. My main relief was sinking into bed—and I usually slept like a rock.

But starting in 2010, something was different. I shifted in bed and couldn't get comfortable. No matter how hard I tried, I couldn't find a position where some part of my body didn't hurt. My hips and collarbone ached, too. I remember thinking we must need a new mattress.

Soon after, I felt like I had the flu. I couldn't shake the feeling that I was dragging, and the fatigue was beyond anything I had ever experienced. I went to the doctor several times complaining of aching and extreme fatigue, but nothing turned up on any of the tests. I just knew something was wrong. Since my mother had thyroid issues, I suspected that could be my problem. I kept hoping something would turn up so I could get relief—some medicine that would help me feel better.

I had more tests and still nothing. I would go to the doctor and cry, trying to explain the amount of pain I was in and the fatigue I was experiencing. I started to do research and became convinced I had a thyroid issue. My doctor insisted I was within normal ranges, but I found that hard to accept. I knew it wasn't normal to feel the way I was feeling. After more research, I came across the ranges used by endocrinologists. According to those ranges, I did, indeed, have an issue. Rather than contact the same doctor who had told me I was "within normal ranges," I made an appointment with an endocrinologist. Sure enough, I was hypothyroid and actually needed quite a large dose of medicine to become regulated. I felt relieved and thought I would get better.

Unfortunately, my symptoms worsened but in a different way. I was still very tired and was constantly sleeping on the couch. But I began to experience more excruciating pain than ever before. I would wake up at night with pains deep in the muscles of my arms—so deep and painful that I would cry. I'd ask my husband to squeeze my arms as hard as he could because that pain was better than the pain that was deep in my muscles. It was so intense that it made me feel like throwing up. Tears would just roll down my face. There was no relief. Because my nights were so awful, I was afraid for the night to come.

Days were better, but not by much. The pain became so intense in my arms that they literally stopped working, making it impossible to do simple tasks like getting dressed and blow-drying my hair. My jaw ached so badly that it was difficult to eat. Sometimes when I'd be sitting my leg would stop working, and when I'd get up, I'd limp. I remember yelping in pain when a teacher shook my hand at a parent-teacher night!

Then, the stiffness began. By January 2011, it became difficult to turn my head when I was driving. When I'd get out of the car, my legs would be so stiff they wouldn't work properly. Things worsened, and I couldn't lift my head off the pillow to read the alarm clock. Even simple tasks were becoming impossible. I couldn't put my clothes on or tie my shoes. My pain was also worsening; I was very scared. I tried taking pain pills left over from prior foot surgery, but no pill could alleviate the pain I was feeling. I understood how people in such pain could no longer go on living. Life was just too unbearably painful. I didn't even feel like eating because nothing was enjoyable. All I could do was lie on the couch in the least painful position. My husband and children were worried, and my husband had to take on the majority of tasks we both used to do. Thankfully, he always believed me and never made me feel bad about not helping at home or participating in the kids' activities. I had a flexible job as a realtor which I loved, but unfortunately, most people there thought I was slacking off, just choosing not to work hard. Because I couldn't get up and had no desire to eat, I lost weight and didn't look well at all. Some people at work were concerned that I had an eating disorder.

Soon after, my wrists started to ache, and I had trouble lifting things. I would take cold packs out of the fridge and put them on my wrists to get some relief. I went back to the doctor and explained what was happening. It was hard to explain without crying because I was in such pain, exasperated and losing hope. I was told *again* that my tests looked fine. I'm pretty sure the doctor thought

I was a hypochondriac. I had such a mix of symptoms that I can see how it might have looked like I was making things up. Aches, pain, fatigue, sore wrists, arms that won't go up, legs that stiffen and cause me to limp. Would I ever get the help I needed?

It was hard to take care of myself, or to do much research because I couldn't sit comfortably for even a short amount of time; I was so tired I couldn't concentrate. I started researching online whenever I could, and things finally clicked when I added "wrists aching" to my myriad of symptoms. It seemed to me like I had an autoimmune disease called rheumatoid arthritis. I had all the symptoms and hoped that if I could discover what I had, I would find relief.

Since my general practitioner hadn't really listened to me or even suggested I see an endocrinologist or rheumatologist, I decided to seek help elsewhere. Having originally come from New York City, I felt that the quality of care was better there. In May 2011, I decided to consult a doctor at the Hospital for Special Surgery—a renowned New York institution with doctors who are experienced in diagnosing and treating rheumatologic conditions. By now, in addition to my other symptoms, the balls of my feet were hurting, and every limb ached. Except for one knuckle on my left hand, I didn't have the typical RA disfiguration. But I had every other RA symptom plus a few others—like deep muscle pain—that were not usual RA symptoms.

My sister and her husband live in Connecticut, so I made the trip there. My sister agreed to go with me to see the doctor. I told my family I was sure I had RA and was confident I would finally be heard!

I was actually looking forward to seeing this doctor because I thought I would get the relief I had been seeking for over a year. I was excited and happy. I greeted the doctor with a smile and told her everything. She looked at me and took both of my hands in hers. She was looking for more typical RA symptoms, and I actually looked better than usual that day. I told her about my symptoms and my pain and how I felt the doctors weren't listening to me. I will never forget what she said: "You do not have RA; you have fibromyalgia. You need to exercise and take better care of yourself. With more rest, better food and exercise, you'll be fine." My sister smiled and looked relieved. She had known a few people with RA and knew what it could do to a person. She was glad to hear that I didn't have it.

I was flabbergasted and upset. "I have something else—I know it," I said. "My wrists are killing me, and I can't lift anything. This is *not* only fibromyalgia!" I thought, "Here we go again. When will someone really hear me?" The doctor shook her head, sighed and said, "Get a sonogram," as if I were wasting her time and the hospital's resources.

My sister and I went down and waited for the sonogram. I was brought into a room where a gel-like substance was put on my wrists, and the doctor began moving an instrument along my wrist area. The doctor and his assistant kept looking at the screen. They were going back and forth and seemed to be very interested in what they saw. One said, "You need to go back up and see the doctor. You have serious erosion in both wrists."

As much as I didn't want to hear that, I finally felt like *now* someone might actually take me seriously. I went back up, and the doctor said, "Oh, you are my mystery patient; you don't look like you have RA, but maybe you do." This, from a person who deals with autoimmune diseases and should know that many people with these conditions don't look like they are ill—something which is extremely frustrating for people with autoimmune diseases! The doctor then directed me to have blood work done. They drew about seven vials.

My results were emailed to me. The diagnosis was "lab work consistent with rheumatoid arthritis." The ultrasound showed that I had inflammatory synovitis in both wrists with bony erosion and marked hypervascularity—meaning cartilage and bone destruction leading to deformity, joint pain and loss of function.

As much as the diagnosis was upsetting, at least I finally knew what I had. I went with my husband to see Dr. Carlos Martinez, a rheumatologist in my area, and he was kind, compassionate and understanding. He gently explained that I had aggressive RA and would need medication to function. He told us about the possible side effects, and I remember sobbing as I sat in his office, confused and in pain, worrying about taking toxic immunosuppressants. I left and filled the prescription for methotrexate, a chemotherapy drug often prescribed by doctors for autoimmune diseases. But I simply could not bring myself to take it.

I began researching RA treatments online. I had long been interested in alternative medicine and had seen the benefits of it with my husband's remission from cancer. I came across an online group for people with rheumatoid arthritis and read whatever I could get my hands on. Finally, I came upon a treatment called Low Dose Naltrexone. I found information about it on Dr. Joseph Mercola's website,[90] as well as on the Low Dose Naltrexone site managed by Dr. David Gluck and his son, Joel.[91] After all my reading, I became convinced that I could benefit from using LDN.

I was not at all impressed and was even disappointed in the doctor I saw at the Hospital for Special Surgery. Still, I followed up with her because I thought perhaps she might prescribe LDN for me. She turned me down, however, telling me that she couldn't help me with LDN because it is a narcotic. (It is not.) I left knowing I had wasted my time and money yet again.

Even though I liked Dr. Martinez very much, I decided to see another rheumatologist even closer to my home. When you're in terrible pain, distance matters. But this doctor also said she could not prescribe LDN because she was not allowed. That's not true, either. LDN is an off-label medication, and all doctors are allowed to prescribe it.

I went back to Dr. Martinez in August 2011 and asked him again if he would prescribe LDN for me. Once again, he was kind and gracious and made me feel like I was his only patient. This time, I gave him the information I had printed out from the Internet, attesting to LDN's success with many patients with autoimmune diseases. He promised to read it and get back to me. Four days later, he called. He had read the information and said, "You seem like a smart young lady, and I don't see any reason why you cannot try this. I only ask that if it doesn't work for you, you will consider traditional treatment." I agreed and thanked him profusely.

Dr. Martinez had his staff send me a prescription. I originally had it filled at a local compounding pharmacy, but as I read more, I decided to have it filled by one of the pharmacies recommended on the LDN website: Skip's Pharmacy in Boca Raton, Florida. I spoke with Skip, and he totally understood LDN, since he has been successfully using it for years himself. I later found out that Skip also has rheumatoid arthritis and has been asymptomatic for many years, thanks to LDN.

There are various suggestions about taking LDN (many suggest gradually working your way up to 4.5 mg), but after about five days on 3 mg, I went directly to 4.5. I had *no* side effects, not even vivid dreams. A few months passed, and I had no relief and was feeling very disappointed. I had lost a year of my life with this disease and was feeling tired, in pain, and hopeless. I was ready to go on the traditional immunosuppressants and made an appointment with Dr. Martinez. I was thinking that maybe I could take LDN and methotrexate together, but I was unsure. I decided to call Skip and ask his opinion. He explained that it's best not to take these two medications together and to hang in a little longer with LDN. (I'd been on it about four months.) I decided I would do that and take prednisone and diclofenac—an anti-inflammatory—as needed, but not methotrexate.

I can't really say what happened as the process was so gradual, but one day I realized I could turn my head to see if a car was coming. Not long after that, I could lift my head to see the alarm clock. My aches in my arms went away, and my legs became less and less stiff. My fatigue and pain lessened, and my jaw no longer ached. I was able to go back to work and resume my usual activities. By the end of 2012, I was feeling much better.

2013 was a good year. My family noticed that I wasn't lying on the couch all the time. I was still very tired, but with a full-time job, my then-16-year-old triplets and a busy family, I guess that was to be expected!

It's been almost seven years since I started LDN. Things are basically the same, except that I no longer need to take diclofenac. I don't think I'm as peppy as I once was, but that could be because I've gone through menopause, or just that I'm older. The triplets—two girls and a boy—are now in college. Their first semester, both girls were homesick. Even though it was a three-and-a-half-hour drive for me to their school in Ohio, I'd often go to have lunch with them and come back the same day. I think I've made at least eight one-day trips like that to see them.

All this time, I've been working full-time. As a matter of fact, I am in the top 10 percent of realtors in western New York State. I take care of the house and live a normal life. I could never have done all this before LDN. Nothing else worked like LDN.

I am so grateful to LDN and to Dr. Martinez, who was the ONLY doctor who actually took the time to listen to me. Thanks to him and LDN, I am a better wife, mother, friend, and worker. LDN has given me back my life.

I have communicated with hundreds of LDN users, and to my knowledge, Maureen's experience is highly unusual in that she found LDN just two years after she began feeling the effects of rheumatoid arthritis. A dramatic difference from all of the people featured in Honest Medicine—*and the other contributors to this book—who struggled for so many years before finding LDN.*

Contributors with Multiple Conditions

CHAPTER 15

Monica Hovden, Norway, Crohn's Disease and Fibromyalgia

Monica Hovden was born in Oslo and now lives in a small town in the southwestern part of Norway. She has struggled with irritable bowel issues since childhood. She was officially diagnosed with fibromyalgia in 1995, and with Crohn's disease in 2001. Monica wanted to share the story of her experience with Low Dose Naltrexone.

Here, in her words, is her story.

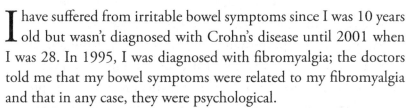

I have suffered from irritable bowel symptoms since I was 10 years old but wasn't diagnosed with Crohn's disease until 2001 when I was 28. In 1995, I was diagnosed with fibromyalgia; the doctors told me that my bowel symptoms were related to my fibromyalgia and that in any case, they were psychological.

At the time when I was diagnosed with Crohn's disease, I was studying to become a healthcare worker. I had lost eight kilos (almost 18 pounds) and needed to use the bathroom up to 18 times a day. In March of that year, doctors finally recommended that I have a colonoscopy and a gastrointestinal endoscopy, and while I was waiting for these tests, I lost another 10 kilos (22 pounds); I weighed only 34 kilos (75 pounds).

The tests revealed massive inflammation in 85 percent of my digestive tract, all the way from my esophagus to my rectum. Doctors put me on high doses of cortisone, as well as iron pills and B12 injections. After three months I felt a little bit better. They then gave me Imurel—an immunosuppressant—intravenously. I experienced many side effects from this medication, including fever, rashes, low blood pressure, and blisters in my mouth.

In late 2001, I decided to try a more holistic approach—a more natural method of treatment—so I went to the Balder Clinic in Oslo. There I was given the highest possible dose of a natural medicine called Moducare, along with a supplement called Synergy. https://www.thesynergycompany.com/pure-synergy. Three to four weeks after starting these treatments, I experienced a reduction in pain and my number of visits to the toilet. After another two months, I was able to finish school and start working again.

Six months later, in 2002, I consulted again with the doctors at the conventional hospital. They made it clear that they had no faith in this more holistic treatment I was using. In fact, they made me sign a document saying that they didn't agree with the treatment and that I was taking responsibility for it. I signed the paper; I wanted to continue with the Moducare and Synergy.

My next checkup, in March 2002, showed that the inflammation in my bowel was reduced. I had started out with 85 percent inflammation. Now I had 35 percent inflammation. This proved to me that the natural treatments were working. In fact, the conventional doctor who looked at the test results had to admit that whatever I was doing was working. He was so curious about these treatments that he called the Balder Clinic to get more information about them.

I continued on this protocol for two years until Moducare was taken off the market. I have no idea why it was taken off the market; it is now back. (The Synergy, though still on the market at the time, was too expensive for me to continue taking it.)

While I was unable to get the Moducare, the conventional doctors put me back on cortisone, as well as on an antacid and painkillers. Even on these medicines, I still had pain and frequent toilet visits—anywhere from 5 to 10 times a day. I lost weight again and didn't feel at all well.

Altogether, until March 2014, I had 10 different treatments lasting for up to two months each. Nothing worked. The low doses of two different chemotherapies were the worst. They caused terrible side effects, including extreme nausea and hair loss. In addition, my liver function was high.

After the last round of chemotherapy, I gave up all hope that any conventional medicines were going to work, and I begged doctors to perform a colostomy (stoma). This is a surgery that creates an opening in the intestine, so feces can bypass the rectum and drain into an external pouch. I was simply unable to handle any more pain and/or take any more sick leave from either of my jobs as a healthcare worker or assistant in a clothing store. I thought a stoma would be my only option.

Another colonoscopy was performed in August 2014. They said I had an inflamed bowel, and that they would consider giving me a stoma. However, in November, they turned down my request for a stoma, because they wanted to try Remsima, a monoclonal antibody medication that was starting to be used for Crohn's disease.

But Remsima didn't work either, and as a matter of fact, I became ill with the side effects, including edema (swelling), hair loss, fever, headaches, and numbness in my legs and arms.

I had had it with conventional medicine!

In early 2015, I learned about the Norwegian LDN documentary, as well as about the Norwegian LDN Facebook group, from a friend who had used LDN successfully for her fibromyalgia. Many people in the group were telling about their successes with this low-dose, off-label drug, for all sorts of conditions, including multiple sclerosis, Crohn's disease, and fibromyalgia. So, in February 2015, I asked my family doctor to prescribe LDN for my fibromyalgia pain. I knew that he wouldn't prescribe it for Crohn's, because he still wanted to give me other conventional medications for it, but I thought he might be open to prescribing it for my fibromyalgia. He refused, saying that LDN was a placebo for hypochondriacs. I told him I had done a lot of research online, but he still refused.

In March 2015, I was still having acute pain and frequent bowel movements and had to take a two-month leave of absence from my two jobs. So, I visited the doctor again. This time, I managed to see a resident physician. I asked him about LDN, and he said that he didn't know much about it, but—although he had not seen the documentary—he knew that LDN existed. He said he would prescribe it if I insisted. He wrote me a prescription for 3 mg tablets. Quite honestly, I had few expectations.

I started taking LDN at the end of March. I had headaches and strange sleep for the first three days, so on the fourth day, I reduced the dose to half a tablet. On the eighth day, when my alarm woke me, I sensed that something was not normal. I had NO pain in my stomach, and I didn't have to run to the toilet before fully waking, which I always had to do before!

I was so happy! I went to work, and everybody noticed that something was different. I was no longer in pain, and I felt like a new woman. I was enjoying life to the fullest. I prayed it would last.

The next few days were wonderful; I was so happy I cried. The improvement continued. Now, my pain is minimal. I have a maximum of two or three bowel movements a day and have not had to take any sick leave. Tests show that I have made vast improvements.

Six months after starting LDN, I noticed that my fibromyalgia pain was also greatly reduced. The truth is that because my Crohn's disease caused me so much pain and inconvenience for so many years, I didn't pay much attention to my fibromyalgia. But after six months of being on LDN, I couldn't help but notice. Throughout the years, I often had to take Pinex Forte, a medication that contains opiates, especially for my Crohn's, but also for my fibromyalgia. Now, since starting LDN, I take only non-opiate pain medications, and I take them only when I have a headache.

Now I have a great life, and I can do my work much better. Still, there are periods when I am fatigued, but it is just wonderful to have a healthy stomach, and not have to spend my working day in the bathroom. Everybody around me notices a huge difference.

My doctor now prescribes LDN and has apologized to me. I guess he sees how well it is working. But surprisingly, even though he sees that I am 100 percent better, he *still* doubts that it is LDN that has helped me. But there is no doubt in my mind. I have a great life, thanks to LDN.

Monica was able to avoid a colostomy, get rid of chronic pain, and put her Crohn's disease symptoms into remission quickly by using LDN. Her fibromyalgia symptoms have lessened, too, although her Crohn's disease has always been her major complaint. Like other patients who tell their stories in this book, Monica had to run a gauntlet of medical opposition before she was able to find a physician to prescribe LDN for her. NOTE: She now uses what is called "alternative dosing" by other members of the Norwegian LDN Facebook group: She takes 3 mg one week and 1.5 mg the next.

CHAPTER 16

Renée Foster, Fibromyalgia and Chronic Fatigue Syndrome

I met Renée Foster on Facebook, where she was the founder of one of the most popular LDN groups, "Got Endorphins? LDN." When I learned her dramatic story about how LDN changed her life after 20+ years of pain from fibromyalgia and debilitating exhaustion from chronic fatigue syndrome, I knew I wanted to include her story in this book. Hers was one of the first contributions I received.

Here is her story.

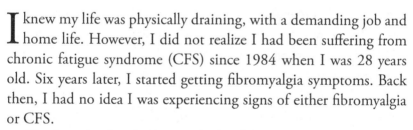

I knew my life was physically draining, with a demanding job and home life. However, I did not realize I had been suffering from chronic fatigue syndrome (CFS) since 1984 when I was 28 years old. Six years later, I started getting fibromyalgia symptoms. Back then, I had no idea I was experiencing signs of either fibromyalgia or CFS.

Thinking back, I had never had a full night's sleep during my whole adult life. My body was stiff and sore. In the beginning, it was mainly my knees, lower back, and upper shoulders. I used to have to force myself to concentrate, or I wouldn't be able to do the tasks at hand. For years, I had been a meat cutter, so I worked with knives and band saw blades. As far back as 1989, I was so brain fogged that many times, I had to talk myself through the steps at work. It was scary. I know now it was brain fog, but back then, I had no idea what was wrong. I was fatigued and tired all the time. I really thought everyone's life was as hard as mine was—that everyone had the same problems: brain fog, fatigue, stiffness, and the inability to sleep.

Being a workaholic all my life, I stayed busy and worked hard throughout much of my illness, both at home and at work. I see now that I was just scared to slow down or sit still for too long for fear I wouldn't be able to get back up. My job as a retail meat cutter was very demanding physically. I was one of the first women with that job in the early 1970s in my district in Southern California. After my apprenticeship, I mostly managed meat departments or was an assistant manager. It was extremely stressful—perhaps, even more so, because I was a woman and some of my co-workers were not happy to have a woman working alongside them!

In 2004, toward the end of my meat cutting career, my health made it necessary for me to go part time. I did some "manager relief" work when a local manager would go on vacation. It was sometimes very challenging to go into a new store and run the department as a manager for a week or two when I had never been inside that store before. By the time I would get the routine down, I would have to go on to the next store's meat department. It was often stressful!

In 2005, after over 20 years of being ill, I was forced to retire from meat cutting entirely at the age of 49. I could no longer keep up with the work because of my health. (Before that, I only took time off from work for two years after my daughter was born in 1991.)

So, I moved into commission sales for a while, working from home. I became very good at it. Being a workaholic, I sat at the computer all day long, making phone calls, and all night, doing paperwork and emails. The stress of working during spring and summer (i.e., the company's "peak season") 15- to 18-hour days eventually became too much for me. Soon I was forced to retire from work entirely.

Still, I wasn't sure why I was feeling so ill—or what exactly was wrong with me.

Then, in 2006, 22 years after my first symptoms began, I came down with a horrible flu. I became ill with flares that wouldn't stop. I was stiff and sore all over, and my whole body was tender to the touch. I was so exhausted that it was almost impossible to get out of bed. I was the mother of a teenager. I love being a mom, so I forced myself to do things for my daughter. I would try my best to do my "mom duties," but I would have to go back to bed after taking her to school. Then, I would wake up to pick her up from school. The same thing would happen when it was time to fix a meal. I would get up, but then, I'd have to be back in bed by 8 p.m.. I was unable to grocery shop, so I did my shopping online. Thank goodness for the Internet!

I could no longer deny that something was wrong. I had no idea what it was—or what I was in for, or how long it would last.

By 2007, I was so ill that I was forced to sleep, stay in bed or sit in a chair for two years! I lived my life looking out a window, hoping for a glimmer of my old self. I had gone from being a person who was lively and productive to being unable to get out of bed or even lift my arms.

That year, I started researching my many symptoms online and concluded that I had had fibromyalgia and chronic fatigue syndrome all along. For years, no doctor was willing to listen or help. Thinking I was depressed, they just kept pushing SSRI antidepressants at me, as well as so-called fibromyalgia meds for my pain. I refused to take SSRIs, or any fibromyalgia meds, such as Cymbalta, Lyrica, or Adderall, to name a few.

Finally, I Learn About LDN!

Daily searching on blogs, forums, and websites kept me going. In the spring of 2010, I found a mention of Low Dose Naltrexone on one website that piqued my interest. I started doing daily searches online, bought some books (*Honest Medicine* was one) and read everything I could find on this immune-system orchestrator. So began more than a year of reading and researching about LDN. I admit I was very skeptical at first, but the more I read, the more curious I became. Once I started reading on blogs and in forums about people who had actually used and benefited from LDN, the more convinced I became that I wanted to try it.

Reading so much about LDN gave me hope. Since there were very few odds against LDN, I was willing to try it.

I soon learned that most doctors are not familiar with LDN and that sadly, they don't care to learn about it. I think there are a few reasons: first, their egos may be involved, and second, many of them don't know how to write a script for a compounding pharmacy. Also, no Big Pharma drug reps are knocking on their doors telling them about LDN. Frankly, LDN is a Big Pharma drug sales killer. For instance, I myself have stopped the regular use of three pharmaceuticals—Vicodin, Ambien, and Ativan—since being on LDN.

I Start Taking LDN.

I asked my doctor about LDN, but he wouldn't even listen. I switched to different medical insurance and asked a few doctors about it. They all refused. Finally, my general practitioner gave me a referral to a pain management doctor. When I called to make my appointment, I told the nurse why I was coming in—that I was interested in getting a prescription for LDN. To my surprise—and to my delight!—when I went for my appointment, I found out that my doctor had actually done research on LDN. Being a pain management doctor, he had used naltrexone in full doses to help patients get off opiates, and one of his colleagues had actually used Low Dose Naltrexone—for fibromyalgia, I believe. He said that at such a low dose, LDN would not hurt me. Since he was new to having medicines compounded, I told him how to word the prescription—"1.5 mg naltrexone, 90 capsules, three refills." He did it. Success!

Within a few days, I noticed that I was slightly less depressed—proof to me that I must have been endorphin deficient for a long time! I thought, "So this is what the real world feels like! I like this feeling!" I started needing Ativan less often for anxiety, and used it only under really stressful circumstances, rather than every day, as before. I was also starting to sleep better and more deeply, the best sleep of my adult life, with dreams I could finally remember. Since I had always been a light sleeper, I did not dream much, only once in a blue moon. Now, I was able to dream again. Thankfully, I was also able to wean myself off Ambien. That drug kept me so groggy all day long and had me getting out of bed to eat at 1 a.m.. I hated it.

I started out low with LDN, at 1.5 mg, and moved up .5 mg each month until I found my best dose—2.5 mg. Within the first few months, my joint pain and osteoarthritis in both knees started to feel 30 percent better, and after a few more weeks, 50 percent better. After I raised my dose to 2.5 mg, I felt 60 to 75 percent better. I continue with that dose to this day. If I go shopping or do house cleaning, or if I have to be on my feet for too long, I may still experience some pain and have to take an occasional over-the-counter (OTC) med. What a great feeling to no longer need handfuls of OTC pain meds every month! NEVER another VICODIN. I am so happy! My immune system saved; my kidneys and liver, too. Not to mention that LDN is inexpensive at the compounding pharmacy I use, and I know they do it right!

During my first months on LDN, my fibromyalgia pain was still there but not as intense; by the fourth month, there was much less pain. To this day, if I sit too long in one spot, I feel some pain and tenderness. However, I am over 60, so that happens to most people at this age, doesn't it?

In 2011, after experiencing such great results with LDN, I decided that I wanted to help others to learn about this low-dose, off-label drug that helped me so much, with hardly any side effects. Actually, most of the "side effects" LDN has for me are good ones. For instance, better moods, deeper sleep, and less anxiety. Happy with LDN, in 2011 I started the LDN Facebook group, "Got Endorphins? LDN" (now renamed "LDN Got Endorphins?"). https://www.facebook.com/groups/GotEndorphins

Its membership has grown steadily, and now we have over 20,500 members. New members join each week. Quite an accomplishment! We are a support group for those learning about LDN or taking it for many different conditions.

I am a huge fan of LDN because of the relief/liberation it has given me physically and emotionally. Remember, I had been ill for so long and was unable to get out of bed. Now I have some semblance of a life. This is HUGE for me. I am so thankful. In the past, I was running at only 10 percent of life; now I can be 60 to 75 percent present in my life again. I know it will only get better and better as LDN continues to orchestrate my immune system into a well-tuned machine once again! I am an LDN Woman and proud of it.

Like the other contributors to this book, Renée has become a tireless advocate for LDN. I am honored that she has made me an administrator of her Facebook group. In this capacity, I get to see the increasing numbers of people who request to become members on an almost daily basis.

CHAPTER 17

Katrien Devriesere, Belgium, Myalgic Encephalomyelitis/ Chronic Fatigue Syndrome, and Fibromyalgia

I met Katrien Devriesere when I posted a request for contributions about LDN successes in the Dutch/Belgium LDN Facebook group, "LDN gebruikersgroep Nederland & Vlaanderen" (https:// www.facebook.com/groups/LDNgebruikersgroepNederland).

Manda-Marieke Schuurer, the administrator of the group, told me that Katrien would like to share her story. Manda-Marieke did the initial translation from the Dutch, making my job so much easier, and both women spoke with me on Skype to fine tune Katrien's story. I am grateful to both women.

Here is Katrien's story.

∽

On June 17, 2016, my husband Marc and I were celebrating our fortieth wedding anniversary in our new home. I had recently turned 60, and after two years of hard work, our new house was finally finished. Thirty friends joined us as we sang and danced; we had lots of fun. Everyone brought something to eat.

A month earlier, Marc and I had moved from the top floor of our house to downstairs, and I handled the whole project myself. That same month, my mother moved into a retirement home. My brother, sister and I cleared our parents' house out together.

I was able to do all of this because of LDN. Before LDN, I was as good as bedridden.

As a child I had a lot of infections, requiring many hospital stays. Several times I was even put in quarantine. I couldn't go to kindergarten, because I was always tired and picked up too many infections from being around other kids.

When I was a bit older, I was able to finish primary school despite frequent illnesses and bouts of muscle pain. During all this time, no doctor was able to figure out what was wrong with me.

When I was 12, I came down with a very serious hepatitis infection and was bedridden for two months. After that, the doctor predicted that I would get better, but nothing could have been further from the truth. My exhaustion never passed.

For me, this marked the beginning of my undiagnosed myalgic encephalomyelitis (ME)/chronic fatigue syndrome (CFS) and fibromyalgia. Despite the fatigue, infections, and pain, I desperately tried to lead a normal life. I held summer and weekend jobs and danced in a folk-dance group. No one ever knew how much I was suffering.

In spite of everything, I remained a relatively happy and optimistic person.

When I was 19, I met Marc at the folk-dance group we both belonged to. The next year we married, and the year after that, when I was 21, our first daughter was born, followed ten months later by our second daughter.

Those were particularly difficult years; I really don't know how I managed. When I heard my children call me in the morning, I was so tired—nearly comatose—that I couldn't get up, or even react. I couldn't explain what was wrong with me. But still, no doctor ever took me seriously.

I consulted many doctors and was given many diagnoses. For instance, one doctor diagnosed me with postpartum depression and treated me with antidepressants; another, with Tietze syndrome, and advised me to take magnesium and vitamin B for my inflamed joints. Still, another diagnosed cardiac arrhythmias and treated me with yet another medication. None of these medications had any positive effects, but since I am very sensitive to all kinds of medications, I experienced many adverse effects. In fact, I tend to get all the side effects listed in the informational packets provided for doctors and patients. These doctors all thought I was a healthy young woman. I believe they thought I was depressed or lazy. They told me to exercise a bit more and just do my best.

One Step Further!

After 10 years of seeing mainstream specialists, I found an alternative/holistic doctor who diagnosed me with ME/CFS and fibromyalgia. He managed to improve my immune system with nosodes (homeopathic preparations) and herbal medicine. I tried acupuncture and much more, including lots of nutritional supplements, such as potassium, iron and Vitamin B12—some by injection, others orally. I was also given lots of hormones. In addition, I took long walks, and participated in sports, including cycling. One doctor also advised me to get rid of my amalgam fillings, which I did.

But still, I failed to improve. In fact, I got worse.

In the years that followed, I continued my quest to get better, but nothing helped. In fact, because of all the exercise I was doing, and the fact that I have ME/CFS, I was actually feeling worse. I was a driving instructor and loved my work, but it required a lot of me physically. I still had many infections and was exhausted all the time. I developed problems with my balance, so I had to quit my job. For outdoor trips, I started using a wheelchair.

I saw a neurologist because of my balance problems. He thought I might have MS, but all the tests proved negative. He had no idea why I kept falling over.

Falling asleep was a disaster. I was prescribed a medication for my insomnia that made me feel like a zombie. So, I tapered that medicine quickly, against the advice of my neurologist. A sleep test in a sleep laboratory showed that I had no REM sleep, and therefore very little deep sleep. One Trazolan tablet—an antidepressant—taken before bed helped me to sleep a bit better.

But still, overall, I didn't feel any better.

For years I was given intravenous drips of magnesium and vitamin C twice a week. It helped a bit in the beginning, but the effect lessened over time.

I began to have more and more problems with my gut, itching, bloating, diarrhea, and leaky gut. An osteopath I'd been seeing for many years treated me for leaky gut and advised me not to eat certain foods (no sugar or lactose; very little gluten) in an effort to heal my intestines. I also took a probiotic.

All this was helpful for my digestion but didn't help with my fatigue, or with my fibromyalgia pain.

In 2002, a professor I was seeing in Brussels, the world-renowned Dr. Kenny De Meirleir, tested me for RNase-L abnormalities. RNase-L (Ribonuclease L) is an enzyme produced by the immune system to defend the body against bacteria and viruses. This test—which is a good indicator of the degree to which someone is sick, especially in the case of ME/CFS and fibromyalgia—came back positive. I don't know why, but after two or three visits, Professor De Meirleir finally gave up on me, saying, "You've been ill for so long; this condition has affected all the cells in your body. There is nothing more I can do for you," and recommended that I lead a quiet life and accept my illness. I cried all the way home from that appointment. My husband, who has always been supportive, saw how I suffered. Even *he* lost hope.

Finally, I Learn About LDN!

In 2014, a friend told me about LDN, a medicine that she and her husband used with success for ME/CFS. I started to read about LDN and became very hopeful that it might help me.

Some Belgian and Dutch websites (the best known was the cutting edge http://www.exendo.be) recommended following an exorphine-free diet (i.e., a diet free of gluten, casein, soy, and spinach) while taking LDN. The rationale: A poorly functioning endorphin system, described as "endorphin resistance" is associated with various health issues. Since LDN works by balancing the endorphin system, exorphines—morphine-like proteins, or peptides, found in foods, such as cow's milk (casein), gluten, soy, and spinach—can undermine that process.

I decided to try the exorphine-free diet, and it worked! My chronic diarrhea disappeared, and the pain from my fibromyalgia lessened. But I still felt ill most of the time.

The osteopath I saw at that time agreed that LDN might help me. He didn't know what else to do to make me feel better. But he insisted that I first get my intestines in excellent condition. However, he was not legally able to write me a prescription, because he was a therapist and not a doctor. [Author's Note: In Belgium, as well as in other countries in Europe, unlike in the US, an osteopath is not considered to be a doctor, and therefore, does not have prescribing privileges.]

In November 2015, after 10 months of bowel treatment and an exorphine-free diet, I was ready to start taking LDN. My friends, who had had such good results with LDN, gave me two 50 mg naltrexone tablets from which to make my LDN. So, from the beginning, I made the LDN myself. I still do. I dissolve half a tablet in a precisely measured amount of sodium chloride 0.9%, which I buy from a pharmacy. This makes the solution last longer than if tap water were used.

After a few weeks, my head felt much clearer, and my energy slowly returned. I also felt less pain. I could do so many things I hadn't been able to do for 40 years. These were my first good years—ever! I was so happy that I sang all day long. Nothing before had helped me as well as LDN. I even went on a trip to Brussels with our grandchildren by public transportation without using my wheelchair for the first time in 20 years!

When my first homemade LDN solution was finished, I decided to convince a doctor to write me a prescription for 50 mg tablets, from which I would continue to make my own LDN. (NOTE: In some European countries, doctors are more likely to prescribe 50 mg tablets, which are not off label, than they are to prescribe Low Dose Naltrexone, which is off label. In addition, in some countries, insurance companies will, therefore, cover the cost of naltrexone, while the cost of Low Dose Naltrexone will not be covered. Some holistic doctors will prescribe actual Low Dose Naltrexone prepared by specialized compounding pharmacies, but many patients find it too costly to go to these doctors.)

I talked to our family doctor in Belgium about it. Like most doctors, she knew nothing about LDN but was willing to prescribe naltrexone for me because she knew about my 30-year struggle to get better. She said, "I suppose you know what you're doing!" and gave me a prescription for 50 mg tablets.

Again, almost immediately after my first day of taking LDN, I felt better: more energy, less brain fog, better memory, less pain. My GP, who had given me the prescription, was shocked when, after around three months, I walked into her consultation room so easily and without pain.

As I write this, I'm taking 1.68 mg of LDN per day. I've tried to increase it several times, but my attempts have all failed. Finding your optimal dose of LDN is a matter of trial and error. As I have found, higher is not always better.

At one point, I had a huge relapse because, after starting LDN, I felt like I no longer had any limits, so I overdid it. I put my wheelchair aside, planned trips, went to parties, and we moved our house. It was just too much, too fast. Also, I was exercising too much after a long period of leading an inactive lifestyle, and this caused a severe hernia. I couldn't sleep for three weeks because of the pain. My muscles were too weak to keep my vertebrae in place. At the same time, I tried to taper my use of Trazolan, the antidepressant I had been taking to help me sleep. That didn't help either.

Whenever I do too much, I have relapses. This is referred to in the literature as post-exertional malaise, or PEM, which is defined as "a worsening of many ME/CFS symptoms as a result of physical or mental exertion. Patients, ME/CFS organizations, clinicians and researchers that work in the ME/CFS field often referred to it as 'the marker,' i.e., the main symptom that differentiates ME and CFS from other fatiguing illnesses. PEM can last for days to weeks after the exertion." http://me-pedia.org/wiki/Post-exertional_malaise

But in general, I feel much better. I still experience fatigue, but when I am fatigued, I don't feel as sick as I used to. I now have more periods of increased energy, much less brain fog, and less pain. In addition, my blood pressure had always been low, and the more tired I was, the lower my blood pressure was. With LDN, my blood pressure has normalized. I have learned that I need to monitor my boundaries carefully.

I'm not cured, but I've restored my quality of life to a great degree. I look completely different: The dark circles under my eyes are gone, and I'm much more energetic. I get so many compliments from people since I've also lost 18 kilos (almost 40 pounds)! I have a social life again, and I can do housework. I even started taking Spanish lessons once a week; I do yoga once a week, too. These things were impossible before because I had such a bad memory and couldn't sit on the floor or get up without help. Now I meditate every afternoon and feel like "me" again.

When I was 52, most of my thyroid, except for two small pieces, was removed because it was full of nodules. After that, I had to take 175 mcg of thyroid medication every day to replace the thyroid hormone my body could no longer make. Since starting LDN, I've been able to lower that dose to 100 mcg. I wish I had known about LDN before the operation. Maybe it could have saved my thyroid and helped me with all my infections.

LDN has done wonders for me. It has transformed my life!

I am very grateful to Katrien for sharing her amazing story. She shares her success with LDN with everyone she feels might benefit from using this life-changing treatment.

CHAPTER 18

Darlene Nichols, Lupus and Myasthenia Gravis

I first learned about Darlene Nichols while searching online for people with lupus who were being helped by LDN. Darlene's story was poignant, but not particularly unusual, in that she went for fourteen years with horrible symptoms and no diagnosis. Also, after being diagnosed with lupus, she went another twenty years before finding LDN.

Darlene was finally diagnosed with lupus in 1989. Ten years later, in 1999, she was diagnosed with myasthenia gravis, another very serious autoimmune disease. But, as you will learn from Darlene's story, she wasn't to find out about LDN until 2009—20 years after her initial diagnosis, and 34 years after the onset of her symptoms. That's when her life truly changed for the better.

Darlene wants to share her story with as many people as she can, in hopes that other people with lupus—and other autoimmune diseases—won't have to suffer the way she did for as long as she did.

Here is Darlene's story.

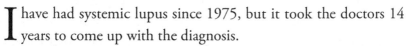

I have had systemic lupus since 1975, but it took the doctors 14 years to come up with the diagnosis.

My husband and I built our first house in 1974, after he got out of the service. We had our second child there. I believed in staying home to raise my children. I wanted to be active in their lives at home and school.

But being an active parent was difficult for me. Every morning, when my husband went to work, I would wake up and try to take care of my six-year-old and my baby.

My problems started in 1975, after the birth of my second son. Before his birth, I hadn't had any symptoms. I was very involved in sports, energetic and healthy. While I was pregnant, I even helped my husband build our house. But starting six months after my son's birth, at least once a week, every week, I would feel like I had a virus. I felt ill, like I had a 102° fever—but I didn't have a fever. I had fatigue that was so debilitating I'd often have to go to bed for the entire day. Still, I'd spend my days trying to take care of the kids and resting when both were napping or, in later years, when they were at school. Every time I'd try to do anything out of the ordinary, like cleaning cabinets or something strenuous, I'd feel sick and have to stop, or I'd become so weak that I'd have to lie down. At other times, I'd do nothing and still wake up feeling ill the next day.

This feeling of sickness never went away for long, so I finally went to my doctor to see what was wrong. At first, he would tell me it was a virus. But, after a few times of seeing him, he finally said he didn't know what was wrong with me, but that a person can't have that many viruses that often!

This went on for at least 10 years. My doctor sent me for all kinds of tests: to a neurologist for an EMG and nerve conductions studies. I was also tested for seizures, heart abnormalities—everything under the sun. But not for lupus! To this day, given my symptoms, I am puzzled as to why I wasn't tested for lupus. The only thing I can figure is that maybe the tests for lupus weren't good back then. Or maybe not many doctors even knew what lupus was. At least that was my experience.

All the tests came back normal. But still both my doctor and I knew something was wrong. He sent me to a stomach specialist who decided I had irritable bowel syndrome (IBS), and put me on an antidepressant and Metamucil. Every doctor I went to said it must be depression or nerves since they couldn't find anything wrong. So, I continued to try being Super Mom and room mother. I even went to my sons' baseball games, sometimes in 95° weather. Invariably, the next day I would be in bed with a "flare," not knowing why.

My whole family was puzzled. They'd wonder, "What's wrong with Mom?" Each time I'd say, "I'm sick again," they'd ask, "Again?" So, I kept forcing myself to do things. I just would not give in to the sickness I was feeling. I cried a lot when I was alone but tried to put on a "brave face" when other people were around. I can also remember eating a lot at fast food restaurants with the kids as my husband worked the evening shift, and most nights I couldn't cook or get dinner on the table. My poor husband didn't know what to do. He was busy working a lot of overtime hours to support us and couldn't be home much, plus he didn't know what was wrong with me. So, looking back, I guess it was a confusing time for him, too.

I think my first lucky break came around 1988. My doctor moved, and I went to a new doctor, an internist, who promised to find out what was wrong with me. First, he changed my thyroid medication as I'd had low thyroid since I was 15 years old. But that didn't do anything for me. So, he sent me to an allergist, who did blood work and said I had "something wrong" with the connective tissues, or vasculitis of some kind. He sent me to a neurologist.

Hearing the words "connective tissues" from the allergist definitely caught my attention. I know this may sound weird, but even before I got the diagnosis, I began to have a "sixth sense"—*a feeling*—that it was lupus. I had done some reading in a magazine about lupus and recognized the symptoms. So, I decided to go to a local lupus support group meeting. It was an eye-opening experience. These people had symptoms like mine! I really felt like God was leading me to them for a reason. They were wonderful and gave me a lot of support.

A week after I attended the support meeting, I went to the neurologist my allergist had sent me to. He did more testing and blood work and finally said, "Well, I'm going to drop the ball on you and tell you that you have lupus," and referred me to a rheumatologist. "Finally!" I said. Even though I had suspected I had lupus, I was glad to get a definitive diagnosis! I went home and told my husband and family. Since, at this point, I had gone to only one lupus support group meeting, we didn't yet know much about this disease or the treatment for it. But we were thankful to get an "official" diagnosis. Most importantly, I was relieved to finally know I was not crazy!

From 1989 until 1993, the doctors treated me with prednisone and other anti-inflammatories, as well as with the antimalarial drug, Plaquenil, which they prescribe for patients with lupus. But nothing worked. When I would get a flare, it would last at least 24 hours, and sometimes two or three days. And nothing could stop it—the fatigue, burning in my legs, legs feeling like they would give out at any time. And one awful thing about Plaquenil is that you need to have your eyes tested once a year, to make sure you aren't developing one of the "side effects" of the drug: blindness! But doctors don't seem to be concerned about this. As recently as 2013, when I was getting my blood work done, my rheumatologist suggested that I go on Plaquenil again! Of course, I didn't do it. [Author's note: It is typical of many LDN patients' experiences that, even after being on LDN for a time, and having virtually no symptoms or disease progression, their doctors still want them to take the "medically accepted," "standard of care" medications—like Plaquenil—even though they are often side-effect-laden and, as in Darlene's case, unnecessary.]

Thinking back, if I'd only had LDN at the time, how different my life would have been. But it was still to be many years before I would learn about this amazing off-label drug.

In the meantime, I found out about another promising treatment from a friend of mine at church who had been diagnosed with prostate cancer. They opened him up to do surgery, said it had spread to his intestines and gave him six months to live. He had heard of Dr. Stanislaw Burzynski, an innovative and controversial cancer doctor in Houston, Texas, and decided to go to him for treatment. There, he learned that Dr. Burzynski would be doing a trial on lupus patients. If I went to Houston, I could get the medicine, antineoplastons,[92] free of charge. So, I thought, "Why not? It's worth a try." I had a family to raise, things to do, and a life to get on with; and the medicines the doctors were giving me were not helping. I didn't have time to be sick!

Dr. Burzynski's FDA trial didn't officially begin until 1996, but he started treating us in his own "unofficial" trial three years earlier. So, in 1993, I began the antineoplaston treatment. Within a few months, I began to feel better. I was still going to lupus support group meetings and told everyone in the group about it. Two of the women there also decided to go to Dr. Burzynski. Four times a year, my husband and I went to Houston for checkups with Dr. Burzynski, as well as for medicine and blood work. (The other two women went separately.) In the following months, every month, the clinic would mail our medicine to us, until our next trip to Houston. At the time, it seemed to me to be a miracle drug: I went into semi-remission.

Dr. Burzynski's treatment worked for me until I began getting symptoms of myasthenia gravis in early 1999. Still, I remained in the antineoplaston trial until January 2002, when it ended—along with the free medicine. In 2002, the FDA stepped in and said that Dr. Burzynski couldn't continue the trial, so we would no longer be able to get the medicine for free. I am really grateful to Dr. Burzynski. He gave me and my friends the antineoplastons free for eight years: for the three years before the official FDA-supervised trial started, as well as during it—until 2001, when the FDA stepped in and stopped him from prescribing it. He never charged us anything during all that time. And my friend who took the antineoplastons for prostate cancer is still alive many years later.

Unfortunately, as I mentioned earlier, lupus didn't turn out to be my only problem. In early 1999, I also started getting a different kind of flare where I would feel weakness in my arms and hips and not be able to walk because the muscles in my hips were so weak. At times, my arms would be so weak I couldn't lift up a fork to eat. I remember going to my son's graduation from law school that year in a wheelchair because, even though my lupus wasn't acting up because of the antineoplastons, I was getting this new kind of flare and couldn't walk. Life was very difficult.

In 1993, I had started working for a neurologist as a transcriptionist. I trusted him, so when I started getting this new kind of flare in 1999, I made an appointment to see him as a patient. He examined me and told me he thought I had myasthenia gravis, as well as lupus. He had a colleague of his put me in the hospital for tests. The EMG and nerve conduction studies performed at the hospital, combined with his observation of my symptoms, confirmed his hunch that I had myasthenia gravis. [Author's Note: People with autoimmune diseases often have more than one.]

He prescribed Mestinon, a drug often given for myasthenia gravis but, since Mestinon can cause diarrhea, and I have irritable bowel syndrome, too, I had to stop taking it. Through all of this, I must give credit to my parents, who were so helpful. My mother even went to some of the lupus support meetings with me. She helped me cook and do other chores when I became incapacitated by myasthenia gravis flares. At this point, I was no longer having lupus flares, thanks to the antineoplastons. And my father also came down and helped when my husband was working and I was too weak to feed myself.

I had read that removing the thymus often helped people with myasthenia gravis. I was under the impression that Barnes-Jewish Hospital, the teaching hospital associated with Washington University in Missouri, was the only hospital in the area where this surgery was being performed. So that year I went to a top surgeon there, hoping he would agree to remove my thymus. He refused, saying he needed to have a firm diagnosis of myasthenia gravis from *their* physician—not mine—and referred me to the top neurologist there who performed the EMG and nerve conduction studies again. But this neurologist interpreted the results of the tests as being negative and said that, in his opinion, I didn't have myasthenia gravis. He wrote in his notes, "The pattern of symptoms is somewhat confusing and not typical for myasthenia. The diagnostic studies appear to have been equivocal." So, the surgeon would not do the surgery.

Five years later, in 2004, I was diagnosed with a cancerous thyroid tumor. This turned out to be a blessing in disguise. Since I had wanted to have my thymus removed anyway, I asked the surgeon to remove it when she removed my thyroid and she agreed. (This surgeon was at another hospital—not Barnes, where they had turned down my request before.)

Having my thymus removed helped to some degree. My arms and legs weren't so weak, so I was able to walk again, and I didn't have to use a wheelchair anymore. But, it didn't really help me as much as I had hoped it would; I was still getting occasional myasthenia gravis flares, and also started getting lupus flares of weakness and fatigue—again after 2002, when I lost the antineoplastons.

My rheumatologist put me on Plaquenil, and then, because of the bad side effects known to occur with this drug, switched me to Cellcept, which is also supposed to work for lupus. I also took prednisone off and on. But nothing was working. I still got flares once a week or so, and since Cellcept suppresses the immune system, I also began to get a lot of infections, my main side effect from the drug.

As an aside, the neurologist I worked for told me that, when they removed my thymus gland and biopsied it, they found that it had a great deal of "activity." As listed in the results of my biopsy: "The right and left thymus specimens reveal thymic parenchyma with reactive follicular hyperplasia, numerous lymphoid aggregates (with germinal centers) are present, a finding which has been associated with myasthenia gravis. Clinical correlation is suggested." This is technical language for "You have myasthenia gravis!"

He called the neurologist at Barnes and told him, "See, you can have myasthenia gravis without certain tests being 100 percent positive. My transcriptionist is an exception to the rule. She had myasthenia gravis under the microscope when her thymus was removed, just as I had suspected." He wrote about my case in a medical journal article pointing out that sometimes the tests—EMG and nerve conduction studies—might not conclusively show myasthenia gravis and that the only way you can tell definitively is by removing the thymus when symptoms are present.

After years of trying various treatments, I was desperate for some relief from the terrible flares of both lupus and myasthenia gravis. I'd spent too many days in the ER with weakness so bad I couldn't lift my hand to feed myself. I also had chest pains so severe that they felt like a knife was stabbing me. The pains were from pleurisy caused by lupus. I asked God again and again to put me in remission, but it didn't happen for me.

Then in April 2009, I received an email from a friend telling me about Low Dose Naltrexone. Thank God for the web and emails! I read about LDN online and asked my rheumatologist to prescribe it for me. She refused, saying she didn't know enough about it to prescribe it. I found a primary care doctor in my area through one of the LDN patient advocates. This doctor was not accepting new patients, but he let me see his associate, who agreed to prescribe LDN for me as long as I made an appointment to see him once a year.

Within weeks of starting on LDN, my flares from both diseases disappeared. At this time, my mother was moving, and I offered to help. Everyone in the family, including me, figured I would get sick the day after helping, as I usually did after trying to do strenuous and stressful things. I went to her house on Memorial Day and packed, then went back and packed and lifted boxes each day for a week after that, and never got sick. My family couldn't believe it, and neither could I.

This is how LDN has worked for me. It's been remarkable. I've been on it since 2009 and have been in remission ever since with no flare-ups of lupus or myasthenia gravis. I am so thankful that I have a life which is normal now. I feel great; I have so much energy and stamina. I can stand at church when I sing in the choir; before, I had to sit. I'm able to do everything a normal person can do, including some things that I had never been able to do before when I was younger.

I feel so lucky that, when my grandchildren were little, I was able to play ball and go boating with them without paying for it the next day with a flare! I was also able to climb into the bleachers to watch their basketball games. For our 50th anniversary, in 2015, my husband and I went to Hawaii and Vancouver. We walked on the beach in Hawaii, and all around the harbor on Victoria Island. Although it was warm—even hot—I was able to keep up with him. I could never have done this before LDN. Plus, I haven't experienced *any* side effects since I began taking it.

I want to add that I used to have a handicapped placard for the visor on my car. But, in 2011, when the rheumatologist saw how well I was doing, she took it away. Proof that—thanks to LDN—I'm no longer handicapped!

One thing I still don't understand, though, is most doctors. I took LDN for three years before my rheumatologist could finally see how well I was doing and agreed to prescribe it for me herself. At first, she thought it was just for multiple sclerosis and said so. She sent me to a neurologist to be tested for MS. I didn't have MS, so I proved to her that LDN works for both lupus and myasthenia gravis, and not just for MS.

I wish I could get everyone with lupus and myasthenia gravis to try LDN. I've told everyone I meet about it, including old friends with lupus and myasthenia gravis. Some people listen, and some don't. All I can do is keep trying to tell my story to everyone who will listen until doctors finally realize just how good LDN is. Thank God for LDN and for the doctors who care enough about their patients to do the extraordinary!

∼

> *Darlene's inspiring story provides us with yet another example of the tremendous success of LDN. It is also a painful reminder of how patients often suffer unnecessarily from a lack of information about—and access to—this extremely effective, low-cost drug. In her case, Darlene went 34 years as a virtual invalid before finding LDN. This is simply unacceptable.*

CHAPTER 19

Kathy Shew, Psoriasis and Multiple Sclerosis

I first learned of Kathy Shew when she posted "before" and "after" photographs in the Facebook group, "Got Endorphins? LDN," showing how her very serious case of psoriasis was helped with LDN. I messaged her about including her story in this book. She said she would love to tell her story so that she can help others who suffer from this horrible skin disease. As you will see, Kathy suffered from multiple sclerosis (MS) for several years before her psoriasis diagnosis. LDN helped both conditions. She has a fascinating story.

Here is Kathy's story, in her own words.

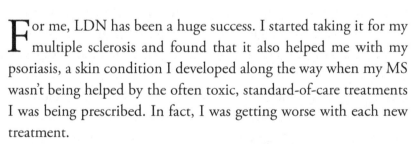

For me, LDN has been a huge success. I started taking it for my multiple sclerosis and found that it also helped me with my psoriasis, a skin condition I developed along the way when my MS wasn't being helped by the often toxic, standard-of-care treatments I was being prescribed. In fact, I was getting worse with each new treatment.

Ironically, I had known about LDN almost from the first day I learned I had MS. My aunt and uncle had introduced me to a woman named Bonnie, who was, and still is, a strong advocate of LDN. She is very grateful for the effect LDN has had on her MS, after having had a terrible reaction to one of the conventional MS drugs. Bonnie tries to tell as many people as she can about LDN.

So, from the beginning, I asked my doctors to prescribe it for me. The first neurologist I met with agreed to prescribe it, but since he said he didn't know anything about it, I foolishly turned down his offer. How I wish I hadn't done that. After him, for many years, all the doctors I approached refused to prescribe LDN. They kept prescribing those toxic drugs which didn't help me at all. I would go six years before finally finding another doctor who would prescribe LDN for me.

My MS probably started in 2009, when I had some numbness in my feet, but I didn't think of it as important. I thought that perhaps my shoes didn't fit correctly, so I didn't consult a doctor. But in 2010, I got up one morning to go to work, and my left hand wouldn't function. I couldn't do anything with it. I freaked out because I thought I was having a stroke. I went to the ER by ambulance, and they did all kinds of tests and procedures—including a CAT scan, MRI, and a lumbar puncture. Everything came back showing that most likely I had multiple sclerosis. The MRI showed lesions on my brain, and the lumbar puncture showed elevated antibodies for an autoimmune process.

I was admitted to the hospital, and they kept me there for a week. They gave me a high-dose IV of a steroid called Solu-Medrol, which had serious side effects for me. It raised my blood sugar to such a high level that nurses had to monitor me every few hours to make sure my glucose didn't become too elevated. In addition, I was in a terrible mood: agitated and angry. These are common side effects of a high-dose steroid. On the plus side, I started to gain function in my left hand by the end of that week. My positive response to the Solu-Medrol helped to convince the doctors that I had MS.

After I was discharged, I shared the information Bonnie had given me with my first neurologist. He basically said, "I would be willing to prescribe it for you, but I don't know anything about it." I thought "What idiot is going to take something when the MS specialist doesn't know anything about it." So, I turned him down. I wish I had said, "You prescribe LDN for me; I'll do all the research." But I didn't.

Thinking back, that was my biggest mistake. Knowing what I know now—and having experienced what I experienced over the past seven years—I wish I had let him prescribe LDN for me.

Instead, he prescribed Rebif, an Interferon that is one of the CRAB drugs. I stayed on it for four years. It kept me stable but affected my skin, since it was an injection, and finding places that were not already bruised from previous injections compromised my skin terribly. After a while, my husband and I had trouble finding spots for the shots. I would get an injection in each upper arm, and then we would do each upper thigh, and then we did each side of my stomach, and then, each butt cheek. We had to rotate the areas, and it got to the point where my skin was all bruised. It was red—inflamed—but I kept getting the injections, and my skin kept getting worse and worse from the shots. In addition, I had to have the shots three times a week, and each time, the day afterward, I would invariably get flu-like symptoms. So, Rebif was problematic.

In 2014, I was prescribed Tecfidera, an oral medication. But Tecfidera gave me stomach issues: nausea, discomfort and, at times, real pain. I stopped that after two months.

Around the same time, in 2014, my uncle noticed that I had a rash on my elbows—dry, flaky and red. That was the beginning of my psoriasis.

This was also the beginning of trying to juggle treatments for two autoimmune conditions, hoping that the treatment for one would not negatively affect the other condition. I would talk to doctors about the side effects of a medication for psoriasis and ask how they thought it might affect my MS, but they didn't know the answer. My dermatologist would refer me to my neurologist, who would say "Well, I really don't know about the skin." Then, my dermatologist would say, "I really don't know about your MS." Sometimes the two specialists would even consult over the phone about a particular medication.

In fact, one time, medication for my MS and treatment for my psoriasis proved to be a dangerous combination.

In May 2015, I began lightbox treatments for my psoriasis, and a few months later, in the summer of 2015, I started taking Aubagio for my MS. That's when the mild psoriasis that had started in 2014 went crazy and spread like wildfire. It got to the point where it was becoming like a body-wide flare. I kept telling my dermatologist that I was getting worse—that I had new spots pop up in different places on my body! But she told me that sometimes things get worse before they get better. I believed her. I didn't think there was a connection. But my psoriasis kept getting worse and worse.

When my neurologist, Dr. G, saw me, she asked, "Are you still taking Aubagio?" When I said yes, she told me to stop taking it immediately; that one of Aubagio's sister drugs, Arava, had been found to make photosensitivity get worse. I had told her about the light treatment before, but at the time, she didn't put two and two together. Aubagio was a new drug on the market, and if you read the information in the booklet that you get with the drug, it doesn't mention photosensitivity. But when she looked at the product information for the sister drug, it mentioned photosensitivity. She finally put two and two together.

In September 2015, I stopped both the Aubagio and the lightbox.

But Aubagio has a long half-life. I had to take another drug, cholestyramine, for around three weeks, to help flush out the Aubagio. Without it, the Aubagio could have stayed in my system for eight months to a year.

Dr. C, my new dermatologist at Hershey Penn State, told me to do a "soak and smear" procedure, followed by applying clobetasol, a steroid ointment. I did fine with this, but when I took a two-week break from the ointment, and my psoriasis came back with a vengeance. [Author's note: Doctors often recommend that patients take a two-week break when using topical steroids, to avoid possible dependence, as well as thinning of the skin and blood vessels becoming more noticeable.]

My dermatologist wanted me to try Stelara. But by now, I was aware that most of these drugs had horrific side effects. She also couldn't guarantee that it wouldn't affect my MS negatively. So, I refused.

I was getting very discouraged. I mentioned LDN to Dr. G, but although she was wonderful in every other way, she refused to prescribe it. She said it wasn't the standard of care, and so, she couldn't prescribe it. In the summer of 2016, Dr. G left private practice to do research at Hershey Penn State.

Although I really liked Dr. G a great deal, her leaving was probably a lucky break for me, because she referred me to Dr. O, a neurologist at Hershey. I asked Dr. O about LDN, and she agreed to prescribe it for me. I was delighted, but not exactly surprised, because Bonnie was going to another neurologist at Penn State—one who was in the same department with Dr. O. So, Dr. O might have heard about LDN that way. I'm not sure. But she wanted me to take a disease-modifying drug along with the LDN. Terrified of the side effects, like those I had experienced with Rebif, Tecfidera, and Aubagio, I refused. But, I did go on LDN.

In September of 2016, I started taking LDN at 3 mg, because that's the dose Bonnie has used for several years. My prescription is filled by Skip's Pharmacy. Nothing happened for six months, but I'm so glad I hung in there and didn't stop taking LDN, because the following March (2017), my skin started to clear. And my MS also stopped progressing. I was feeling better and had less anxiety. I experienced a better mood, more energy, and less brain fog. I have a better outlook on life now, and I can think more clearly. Looking back, I used to be depressed and couldn't focus or concentrate. But six months after I started the LDN, I was feeling much better. In fact, I feel better on LDN than I ever felt on any of the drugs I took for MS or psoriasis.

I haven't seen my dermatologist since I've started taking LDN. I even canceled my most recent appointment, since my skin was doing so much better. And besides, the last time I was there, my skin was so bad that the director of the dermatology department requested that I come to the hospital once a week to be observed by medical students. It's a teaching university hospital and, because my psoriasis was so severe, they wanted me to help their students learn. But I didn't want to be a "guinea pig." Also, I live an hour-and-a-half away, so it wasn't convenient for me to go there every week.

But I truly do want her to see how much better my skin is doing. I'd say that it is now 85 percent clearer than it was when she first saw me. I plan to make an appointment with her soon.

Also, my MS is stable. My neurologist, Dr. O, who prescribed LDN for me, was so happy that my annual MRI a year ago showed no changes. She was also pleased that my skin had improved. When I see her for my next appointment, I know she'll be happy that my skin has improved even further.

At first, I took my LDN at night, before bed, the way most people recommend doing it, but I felt like I was awake while sleeping. So now, I take it at 7 a.m., when I wake up. The fact that taking LDN in the morning is effective for me speaks to the power of LDN.

Kathy's story serves as a warning to people who suffer from more than one chronic condition. As she found out, a medication that is prescribed to treat one condition might very well negatively affect, or even exacerbate, the other condition. In Kathy's case, using LDN made it so that she was able to discontinue the use of her other medications.

CHAPTER 20

Margaret Schooling, France, Rheumatoid Arthritis, a Blood Disorder, a Tumor, and an Eye Problem

I first met Margaret Schooling years ago, when I was creating my first publication about LDN—a free online ebook, titled The Faces of Low Dose Naltrexone. *Margaret offered to transcribe some of the interviews that had originally aired on Mary Boyle Bradley's LDN Internet radio program. I later adapted her transcriptions for two of the LDN advocates' chapters for* Honest Medicine.

At that time, I learned that Margaret herself was a satisfied user of LDN for her rheumatoid arthritis (RA). I tucked this information away in my brain, and approached her years later, and asked her to share her LDN story for this book.

Margaret was born in the United Kingdom but has lived in France for 27 years and now has dual citizenship. She grew up in London and did secretarial work overseas in Europe, Africa, South America, and London. She is a citizen of the world.

As you will see from reading her story, in addition to RA, Margaret also had three other medical conditions—a blood disorder, a tumor, and an eye problem. LDN helped all her conditions.

Margaret shares her story here.

I didn't know anything about rheumatoid arthritis before December 2008, when my GP told me I had it. Three months earlier, I had pain where my hand joins the wrist, and the back of my hand was badly swollen. It was bruised and hurt a lot.

Looking back, I think my immune system had been compromised from an early age. For instance, in my late teens I noticed an enlarged finger joint, my feet were cold and sweaty, and I had night sweats.

My most vivid memory of my first symptoms, before the joint pain began in earnest, was dreadful muscular fatigue. I had to lie down after doing the simplest things: vacuuming, washing my hair, things like that. I had three short courses of prednisone, the third for about six weeks, from January to February 2009. For about a week I felt fit and strong. But it didn't last.

At about the same time as the RA pain began, I noticed a deterioration in my eyes. In 2004, after my second cataract surgery, I was diagnosed with macular degeneration (AMD), but until 2008, I didn't notice any actual deterioration in my eyesight. Suddenly it was blurred and distorted.

By then the RA had spread to the rest of my body, and my feet felt like I was walking on pebbles. The local rheumatologist said it was "polyarthritis," simply meaning that more than five of my joints were affected. He said there was nothing he could do. He prescribed painkillers, but I never took them.

Around February 2009, a friend told me about Dr. Joseph Mercola's article about LDN and rheumatoid arthritis, "Can LDN Really Help Multiple Sclerosis, Rheumatoid Arthritis and Other Autoimmune Diseases?" https://articles.mercola.com/sites/articles/archive/2009/01/13/can-ldn-really-help-multiple-sclerosis-rheumatoid-arthritis-and-other-autoimmune-diseases.aspx

At first, I thought it sounded really flaky, so for about six weeks I researched LDN online, and became a member of several LDN groups. I learned a lot from a forum called Proboards, administered by a woman named Brenda. The group is still going strong and Brenda is still the administrator: http://ldn.proboards.com. I also learned a lot from the LDN Yahoo group, and the information I found on Linda Elsegood's site, http://LDNResearchTrust.org, was extremely helpful, as well. An added benefit: I was able to talk with Linda on the phone. She was very reassuring.

After doing my research, I decided to try LDN. I didn't know if it would help me, but it seemed worth a try. I asked my GP for a prescription, explaining how I'd dilute the tablets and she shrugged, said, "Why not?", and wrote me a prescription for 50 mg naltrexone tablets, which I had filled by a local pharmacist, who gave me a funny look because I didn't look like a drug addict or an alcoholic!

So, on April 22, 2009, I started LDN at 1 mg and increased the dose to 4.5 mg within a few weeks.

I kept a journal for a while. Sometimes I had headaches; sometimes, I felt agitated and angry. And sometimes I felt sick. But sometimes I felt better. No day was like any other. However, on April 26, 2009, I had an amazing experience. First thing in the morning and without thinking, I picked up the kettle with one hand. This was something I hadn't been able to do for a long time. By May, my fingers were beginning to straighten, and the deformities gradually disappeared. Some months later, I could clench my hands again.

By the summer of 2009, my RA was no longer a problem. I began to notice other improvements, too. The first non-joint improvement I noticed was with my eyes. After about three days on LDN, there was less blurring and less distortion. I hadn't expected this; at first, I thought it might be wishful thinking. Although my eyesight isn't as good as it was before I became ill in 2008, I still only need reading glasses.

Another unexpected improvement came with the blood disorder I had been diagnosed with in 1986. At first, they diagnosed me with polycythemia, but now they say it is essential thrombocytosis. Whatever the diagnosis, the fact is that the improvement in my bloodwork was so noticeable at my annual checkup in 2012, that my hematologist agreed to prescribe LDN for me. (The pharmacist gave me 28 50 mg tablets, from which I again made my own LDN. I still do.) My blood tests—three times a year—continue to show that I am normal and stable.

The fact that my hematologist was now prescribing LDN for me was very good news. My GP had prescribed 50 mg tablets of naltrexone for me in 2009. In 2010, however, her partner refused to continue to prescribe it, saying she could get into trouble for doing so. She told me that, in France, a GP can only prescribe a medication that is not recognized by the health system if a specialist has prescribed it first; otherwise, not. So, for two years, 2010 and 2011, I had been buying my 50 mg naltrexone tablets from India. I was glad to be able to get a prescription that I could get filled locally once again. Also, with our health system, I get it for free.

The next year, 2013, however, my hematologist went even further and said I didn't need to see him anymore, that I should keep having blood tests, but only three times a year, and that I should have the results sent to him. He gave me his email address in case I needed his advice.

However, although he gave me that precious prescription, he would not agree that the LDN was responsible. He said it was probably a coincidence.

Since then I've only needed to see my GP once a year for my LDN prescription and blood tests.

On April 1, 2009, my guts suddenly went haywire: a kind of diarrhea set in and continued relentlessly. I went from 60 to 45 kilos (130 to 99 pounds) in three months before I was hospitalized at the end of July, put on drips and given a colonoscopy. The gastroenterologist said they found a small ulcer in my small intestine. He had it biopsied. I was sent home but was back a few weeks later at the end of August 2009 for 10 days, with low potassium and feeling wretched. The gastroenterologist said the biopsy had shown a small benign carcinoid tumor. He thought it might be giving off a hormone that disrupted the liver, causing my diarrhea. He planned to remove that section of the intestine, but first, he had to make sure it had not spread. He scheduled two whole-body octreoscans—a kind of scan used to detect certain types of tumors—for November 2009. I came home, took potassium pills and had regular blood tests to help adjust the dosage.

In January 2010, my gastroenterologist told me that—to his surprise!—there was no sign of any tumor anywhere in my body. I told him I was taking LDN, but he shrugged it off, refusing to see it as anything more than a coincidence. I haven't seen or heard from him since. The diarrhea gradually got better. By October 2010, I was starting to feel normal again. By 2012, my guts were totally back to normal.

I believe the LDN began working on the carcinoid tumor straightaway so that by the time it was found in June, it was already shrinking. It was gone by November.

Although RA seemed to be the start of my problems, I can only think it was the latest manifestation of autoimmune disease, and that the blood problem was there first. It's impossible for me to concentrate on one and not the other. LDN helped with *all* of my problems.

I'm 75 now. I do everything around the house and only need help a couple of times a year to cut the grass. I am very busy with my volunteer work, and I don't need to take any days off. I still drive, and work with several organizations as a volunteer—one in the UK, and the others locally, in France. Most of my work is in the area of history, especially medieval genealogy. I write the newsletter for one of my volunteer organizations and have been treasurer for another for about seven years. I have lived in France for many years, and because I speak French, I'm able to help my compatriots—other British people who have settled in my village—when they need an interpreter. I follow world events and environmental developments, and I sign a lot of petitions.

Physically, I am fine. I see my GP once a year to get a refill of my prescription for 28 50 mg naltrexone tablets, which lasts me a year. At that time, she checks my blood pressure, lungs, and heart. I now weigh about 53 kilos—around 115 pounds. I seem to be more sensitive to insect bites and, at times, I need to take an antihistamine. I think it could be environmental. I have a few other problems, but nothing serious.

I make my own LDN, rather than buying it from a compounding pharmacy, by diluting a 50 mg tablet in 50 ml of boiled, filtered tap water which I keep in a small bottle in the fridge. I draw off the number of ml I need with a needleless syringe and take it at around 9 p.m. every night. Although I can now skip it for a day once a week, I don't envision ever stopping LDN. It has changed my life.

I'm still the moderator of the LDN rheumatoid arthritis Yahoo group. We have around 700 members but very little activity. I'm happier to talk about LDN than others are to hear what I say. Somehow my message isn't convincing. One colleague said she wasn't going to take "any old thing." Two friends who took it after witnessing my response don't take it anymore, even though a prostate shadow disappeared and has now come back. I think people are very loath to disregard or go against what their doctors tell them.

The French LDN Facebook page is gradually becoming better known, and I help there when I can by answering questions.

But in the end, I've opted to work with my favorite subject—history—in my local neighborhood in France.

Margaret's story serves as an inspiration for those who suffer from a combination of conditions, all of which have been helped by LDN.

GOING FORWARD

CHAPTER 21

How to Convince Your Doctor to Prescribe LDN for You

Now that you've finished reading *The Power of Honest Medicine*, you may be asking, "How do I convince my doctor to prescribe LDN for me?"

It's a valid question, and one I've been asked hundreds of times by patients and their advocates who have heard me speak about LDN on the radio.

To help respond to this need, I began offering group teleseminars and individual coaching sessions dedicated to teaching patients how to convince their doctors to prescribe LDN.

I gave my teleseminar attendees and coaching clients lots of tips and materials to share with their doctors—all with the goal of helping their doctors feel comfortable prescribing LDN.

Before I share this information with you, there are a few things you need to know. Specifically: why doctors are not more open to prescribing treatments they learn about from their patients.

Doctors are Trained, not Educated.

In *Honest Medicine*, Dr. Burt Berkson writes that doctors are *trained* and *not educated*. This is key. He points out that training is different from education. Training means listening to the professor, taking notes, and spitting the information back on the test. With this mindset, doctors are open to prescribing only those treatments they learned about in medical school or from their professional journals. That's training, which is rote learning. Education, on the other hand, implies open-mindedness and curiosity. This difference explains a lot about many doctors' skepticism about any unfamiliar treatments you are sharing with them.

There is also the problem of how doctors view the doctor-patient relationship.

Ask most doctors how treatment decisions *should* be made, and you'll usually get one of two answers. Most doctors, especially those from the "old school," expect to tell their patients which treatment(s) *they* recommend. They assume their patients will go along with their suggestions; no questions asked.

Doctors who are more open-minded will *say* they believe in "doctor-patient collaboration." However, what this usually means to them is: The doctor gives the patient a few treatment options, and together, the patient and doctor choose which of *the doctor's options* to pursue. Again, there's no real input from the patient.

With this mindset, the patient cannot suggest a treatment option to the doctor and get a positive response.

But reading this book—and *Honest Medicine* before it—means that you are a different kind of patient: an empowered patient. Empowered patients come to the doctor and say, "I've learned about a treatment I want you to evaluate *with me*."

Unfortunately, many doctors aren't "there" yet. Happily, some are.

Approaching Your Doctor about LDN: Four Steps

There are four steps to take when approaching your doctor about being treated with LDN.

1. Research!

First, do your own due diligence. Read as much as you can and learn a lot about LDN before you approach your doctor. That way, before you ask him or her to prescribe it, you'll know what you're talking about.

2. Assemble the Best Research for Your Doctor.

Next, identify a few key articles and studies that you think will be most persuasive and put them neatly together in a folder designed to make a convincing presentation.

In helping my clients figure out which articles to share with their doctors, I tell them to choose those that are closest to the kinds of scholarly articles doctors like to see.

For instance, I have my clients share this impressive interview with Dr. Bihari from *Alternative Therapies Magazine*. (http://honestmedicine.typepad.com/ldn_teleseminar/Alternative-Therapies_Bihari-reprint.pdf)

In the first few lines, your doctor will learn that Dr. Bihari was Harvard-educated, double-board-certified in neurology and psychiatry and that he ran several New York City programs for heroin addicts. Your doctor will also learn about how Dr. Bihari became knowledgeable about naltrexone, a drug originally approved by the FDA at high doses for treating heroin addicts, and how he discovered that lower doses helped many people with autoimmune diseases. Even though this interview was published in an alternative medicine publication, it will go a long way toward influencing any doctor who is at all open to learning from a patient about a new treatment.

There are also many small LDN studies conducted at prestigious institutions and published in equally prestigious journals. Share these studies with your doctor and, if possible, bring the *whole* studies as originally published, rather than abstracts.

If you have Crohn's disease and want to try LDN, share the three studies performed at Penn State, all of which show LDN to be effective for Crohn's. They were published in the *American*

Journal of Gastroenterology, Digestive Diseases and Sciences, and the *Journal of Clinical Gastroenterology.* You may have to pay to obtain the full articles but, in most cases, you won't have to pay much.

Similarly, if you want to try LDN for fibromyalgia, three studies were performed at Stanford University, published respectively in *Pain Medicine, Arthritis & Rheumatology* and *Clinical Rheumatology.* All showed LDN to be effective.

I have put together abstracts of several of the small LDN studies, as they appear in the government-run database PubMed. You are welcome to share this collection with your doctor. http://honestmedicine.typepad.com/ldn_teleseminar/LOW%20DOSE%20NALTREXONE%20STUDIES%20BY%20DISEASE.pdf

For more complete listings of LDN studies—listings that are frequently updated: https://www.ldnscience.org/research and https://www.ldnresearchtrust.org/ldn-clinical-trials

3. Get Ready to Present Your Information to Your Doctor.

Presentation is important. If you want to have a better chance of convincing your doctor to be your partner in this effort, bring the articles to your appointment neatly in a folder. Say, "Doctor, I've put together some information about a treatment I've been studying for my condition. I'd like to leave it with you and make another appointment to come back and talk with you about it. When do you think would be an adequate amount of time for me to make another appointment?"

Your doctor will either say, "I'm not interested," or will tell you to make another appointment to discuss the treatment in two weeks—or three weeks, or even four weeks. If the response is positive, you've been successful.

An important note. *Do NOT* say, "I found this treatment on the Internet." Or, almost as bad, "I heard a woman on a radio show talk about this treatment." Doctors hate that. It reminds me of my dad, a general practitioner in the 1960s and '70s. Patients used to bring him articles about treatments they learned about in the *Readers Digest*. He hated that. He found the idea that his patients might believe the *Readers Digest* knew more than he did very upsetting.

4. Be Ready for Your "Presentation Appointment."

Once your doctor has agreed to talk with you about LDN, it's important that you do everything you can to make sure the appointment itself goes well.

Be sure to bring a copy of your informational packet for yourself, identical to the one you left with your doctor.

Guide your doctor to the important points in your materials. For instance, point out Dr. Bihari's impressive background, as detailed in the introduction to the *Alternative Medicine Magazine* interview.

When talking to your doctor about the studies, point out the respectability of both the institutions where the studies were performed and the journals in which they've been published. Note, too, the promising conclusions—for instance, conclusions like "significantly improved," "appears effective," "improves clinical and inflammatory activity," "an effective, highly tolerable treatment," etc.

If Your Efforts Fail

Many of my clients have been able to convince their doctors using this four-step approach. Others have not. When this happens, I advise my clients to ask, "If I find another doctor to prescribe LDN, will you still be my doctor, and will you still follow me?" Hardly any doctor has refused to follow a patient who uses this method. In fact, one of my clients calls this question "Julia's magic words."

If your doctor refuses to prescribe LDN for you, don't give up hope. Although it is always best to have your doctor prescribe LDN for you—after all, he or she knows you best!—you can find another doctor who will. Names of LDN prescribing doctors may be found at https://www.ldnresearchtrust.org/LDN_Prescribers and https://www.ldnscience.org/patients/find-a-doctor.

If you don't find a doctor in your state through one of these lists, I recommend contacting LDN patient advocate Crystal Nason at angelindisguiseldn@yahoo.com. Crystal has kept, maintained, and updated, her list for several years now.

Becoming an LDN Success Story

As you can see, presenting information to your doctor about a treatment he or she doesn't know about—like LDN—can be complicated. But, if you have been taking the medications your doctor has been prescribing, with little or no success, you should be ready to follow your gut—your intuition—and start looking for a treatment that might bring you greater relief.

It may not be easy to confront your doctor about a new treatment like LDN—especially when you realize that, at least at first, your request may be met with skepticism or even hostility. Remember, however, that ultimately, your doctor works for you, and that you need to be empowered to make decisions that will help you get well and stay well. This is even more important if you have a chronic and potentially debilitating condition and are not getting relief from medications your doctors are prescribing, or if you are experiencing unacceptable side effects from those medications.

Every one of the people who shared their stories in this book was, at first, afraid to confront their doctors. Most initially met with resistance. But in the end, each one finally overcame fears, became empowered, and ultimately was able to become an LDN Success Story.

You can do it, too. I wish you every success in your health journey!

AFTERWORD

The Media—For Good, and Not So Good

As you learned from reading this book, and *Honest Medicine* before it, I fervently believe that the media plays a powerful role in letting the world know about medical treatments, both valuable and not so valuable—and in some cases, even harmful.

In *Honest Medicine,* Hollywood writer/producer/director Jim Abrahams (*Airplane, Hotshots*) shared his personal story of how he became determined to spread the word about the Ketogenic Diet after it cured his son Charlie of his intractable seizures, literally overnight. Without Jim's understanding of, and access to, the media—in his case, television and film—I am sure that the Ketogenic Diet would never have survived, much less thrived. Because of this, today, many thousands of children with epilepsy are seizure-free. And, just as important, without Jim's championing of the diet through the media, I sincerely doubt that the diet would be used today with such success as an integral part of so many patients' cancer-fighting protocols.

Similarly, in this book, we learn how Frank Melhus, featured in Chapter 5, channeled his delight at how LDN resolved his near blindness caused by optic neuritis into a documentary that aired on TV2, the largest television station in Norway. This documentary became the most watched show in Norway in 2013, and is now on the Internet, with and without English subtitles. The result: Use of LDN in that small country skyrocketed from 300 to 15,000, literally overnight, with 75 percent of general practice doctors being willing to prescribe it.

One of the reasons I am so happy that Frank agreed to tell his inspiring story in this book is that I hope it will encourage other documentarians and producers with access to the media—and success using LDN—to do the same thing.

And we can't ignore online media either.

How many contributors to both *Honest Medicine* and this book uttered the phrase (or variations of it), "Thank God for the Internet!" when, after a long journey through conventional medicine with its many toxic drugs, they finally learn about–and get—the treatments featured in both of these books?

Whether it was viewing Frank's documentary in Norway, or joining online chat groups and forums, the media has been a blessing for people searching for treatments for conditions like those featured in these two books—as well as in similar books.

The media has a very special personal meaning for me. In the Afterword to *Honest Medicine*, I relate how my Grandpa Turitz was told in 1928 by Dr. Charles Mayo (yes, *the* Dr. Charles Mayo!) that my grandmother had six months to live. Luckily, he read a column in his "bible," the *Jewish Daily Forverts*, about a promising experimental treatment in Germany for colon cancer and sent Grandma Julia there. She survived for 11 years, instead of the six months Dr. Mayo had predicted.

This story is part of my DNA—and of my belief in the role of the media in doing good. By the way, my grandmother sent Dr. Mayo holiday cards every year *until he died!* (She outlived him by a few months.)

The Negative Side of the Media

But there is a flip side to this story of how the media influences our treatment choices. It is the story of how the mainstream media, especially in this country, is controlled by Big Pharma, Big

Industry, Big Government, and major medical institutions. All four work together to keep information about successes with unconventional treatments like those I write about *out of the media*, and therefore out of the public's consciousness.

How Mainstream Media Works

An example: As long as Robert Kennedy Jr. was writing about the environment and climate change, he was welcomed as a guest on major television shows, and as a writer of opinion pieces in the major press. However, after the publication of his book, *Thimerosal*, when he started advocating for greater safety in the manufacturing of vaccines (a decidedly anti-big-pharma topic), things abruptly changed. Kennedy was no longer welcome in major—or even minor—television markets. Nor was he able to write opinion pieces for publications like *The New York Times* or *The Washington Post*.

In a May 2015 interview with Jesse Ventura, recounted in Kevin Barry's book *Vaccine Whistleblower*, Kennedy described the power of the media to keep controversial health information out of the mainstream:

> I ate breakfast last week with the president of a network news division, and he told me that during non-election years, 70 percent of the advertising revenues for his news division comes from pharmaceutical ads. And if you go on TV any night and watch the network news, you'll see they become just a vehicle for selling pharmaceuticals. He also told me that he would fire a host who brought onto his station a guest who lost him a pharmaceutical account.

No surprise. Just very well stated.

It's no surprise that a celebrity like Cyndi Lauper appears in a TV ad for Cosentyx, an injectable biologic FDA-approved for the treatment of psoriasis, with side effects such as increased risk of infections. https://www.ispot.tv/ad/wbeh/cosentyx-clear-skin-can-last-2-featuring-cyndi-lauper

When one researches more carefully, it turns out that four people in one Cosentyx study developed malignant melanoma, a virulent form of cancer.

A very serious "side effect," indeed!

Even so, most conventional doctors are more comfortable prescribing a drug like Cosentyx than they are prescribing LDN. In Chapter 19 of this book, Kathy Shew tells how several doctors rebuffed her efforts to be treated with Low Dose Naltrexone. Instead, she was encouraged to use more toxic drugs, like the injectable biologic, Stelara, which has an increased risk for skin cancer. Thankfully, she refused to take Stelara and was finally prescribed LDN. Her psoriasis is now in remission.

Print Publications

When you look at major magazines, a similar picture emerges: a preponderance of pharmaceutical ads, running two, three, and four pages long. Is it any wonder then that a majority—if not all—of the health stories in these magazines are about mainstream medical treatments, and none are about treatments that buck the mainstream medical system? So, while there are lots of stories about cancer, most of the people featured in these stories use the standard of care—surgery, chemo, and radiation, for example—and maybe they add reiki, yoga and a change in diet. But there are virtually no stories about people who buck the standard-of-care treatments and choose treatments like those I write about.

Mainstream Media's Influence on the Treatment of One of the Conditions I Feature in this Book

Parkinson's disease has perhaps the highest profile of any of the conditions featured in this book. Michael J. Fox's heavily publicized efforts to find a cure for his own Parkinson's disease have kept it in the news. In 2000, he created the Michael J. Fox Foundation, which has become the largest nonprofit funder of Parkinson's research in the world, investing more than $650 million in research to date.

Many people in the LDN community who have experienced positive results using LDN for Parkinson's have reached out to Fox to ask him to fund studies using LDN for PD. Their requests have all been ignored.

Strangely, in 2009, the Fox Foundation funded a study of naltrexone (NOT Low Dose Naltrexone, but HIGH DOSE naltrexone) for impulse control disorder (ICD), a condition that is a side effect of some Parkinson's medications. (In her contribution to this book, Lexie Lindstrom described becoming a shopaholic as a result of taking the Parkinson's drug, Requip.)

Ironically—and sadly—the dosage used in the Fox Foundation study of 50 patients was high: 50 to 100 mg. This entirely ignored the work of LDN pioneer, Dr. Bernard Bihari, who pointed out that this high dose—which had been approved for heroin addiction—was incredibly toxic and intolerable for his patients who took it. In his words:

> And when the drug came out, I was interested in trying it. I gave it to about two dozen heroin addicts who had recently stopped using heroin. None of them would stay on it. At the doses involved, it caused anxiety, depression, irritability. They couldn't sleep, and even minor stresses that they could handle the day before, they couldn't handle on days that

they took naltrexone in the morning. So, it was out on the market, and has remained so since, but has been relatively little used.

http://honestmedicine.typepad.com/ldn_teleseminar/Alternative-Therapies_Bihari-reprint.pdf

Not surprisingly, Fox's study, which I am sure was very costly, garnered decidedly mixed—even confusing—results. Results were found to be "negative for the efficacy of naltrexone for the treatment of impulse controls disorders," but concluded that when patients were surveyed they said naltrexone worked better than the placebo. https://www.michaeljfox.org/foundation/grant-detail.php?grant_id=567

WHAT!!??

How I wish Fox had not ignored the pleas from the LDN community to study LOW dose naltrexone, rather than the higher doses. Many of us believe that LDN would have produced far better results. If that had happened, with the publicity that would have resulted, more doctors would now be open to prescribing LDN for their Parkinson's patients. And more Parkinson's patients might well be realizing results similar to those Lexie realized, as she describes in this book.

My Personal Parkinson's Experience

The once-famous photographer Margaret Bourke-White also comes to mind. Bourke-White was the first high-profile person I know of to go public about her battle with Parkinson's. "Famous Lady's Indomitable Fight" was the title of an article and photo spread that appeared in *Life Magazine*, shortly after she underwent a controversial experimental operation—chemothalamectomy—in an effort to alleviate her symptoms. The highly invasive surgery involved drilling a hole in her skull and injecting alcohol into the portion of the brain known as the thalamus. Her neurosurgeon Irving S. Cooper believed that damaging these cells could dramatically improve her mobility.

The operation seemed to work at first, but it's not clear why. The problem is—or was—that while it worked in the beginning, it stopped working, and Bourke-White's condition deteriorated until her death in 1971. (This surgery is no longer being performed. Dr. Cooper, however, went on to become a pioneer in deep brain stimulation, the surgery for Parkinson's that is still being performed today.)

Bourke-White's experience has a very personal significance for me. Shortly after she underwent that surgery, I was a student in a high school that was within walking distance of her home. A friend and I managed to get an interview with her. We planned to write an article for our school's newspaper about her victory over Parkinson's disease, thanks to this experimental surgery. We arrived at her door at the appointed time and rang the bell. We waited—and waited. We rang again and again. After what seemed an endless amount of time, Ms. Bourke-White finally opened the door. Her feet dragged, her face was immobile, and her hands trembled. Obviously, whatever benefits she had first experienced from the surgery had disappeared.

I have no idea—no memory—of how my friend and I endured our "interview." I do remember that Ms. Bourke-White was extremely gracious and that she praised the surgery and her surgeon a great deal. But I think the three of us were all aware that "the jig was up."

It has been many years since my friend and I met Margaret Bourke-White. But this story stays with me as a reminder that some of the "miracle" treatments devised by our conventional medical system can be highly toxic—even dangerous—and they often don't work. And because these treatments are either produced by big pharmaceutical companies, or championed by major medical centers, they benefit from a great deal of publicity in the mainstream media, causing many patients to seek them out, and many doctors to recommend them to their patients. And in situations like this one, I believe many patients have been harmed.

At the same time, a treatment like LDN—and other treatments I write about—*do* work for many people, are extremely safe, and have stood the test of time. Yet, because of lack of money, they don't get coverage in major magazines, like Margaret Bourke-White's *Life Magazine* profile, and they don't have celebrities like Cindy Lauper promoting them. And because these treatments don't get major publicity, they aren't as well-known as they should be. And this means that all the people who could be helped don't get that help.

When will the media start to *really* do its job?

APPENDICES

APPENDICES

APPENDIX A:

LDN Resources

Since *Honest Medicine* was published, information about LDN has ballooned to the point where I refer to this innovative treatment as a *cause célèbre*. There are LDN websites in several countries; many books written about it; conferences held almost every year since 2005 devoted to it; nearly 30 Facebook groups, in the US and abroad; and many online forums and chat groups—all devoted to LDN.

This appendix attempts to list the most important of these resources. By the time you read this, there will, of course, be more. I apologize in advance if I have left any important resources out.

WEBSITES—GENERAL

LowDoseNaltrexone.org and LDNInfo.org

http://www.lowdosenaltrexone.org and http://www.ldninfo.org

Dr. David Gluck's website, created with his son Joel. This is the first LDN website and is considered *the* LDN website. Contains lots of information about studies, compounding pharmacies, and the LDN conferences from 2005 to 2013. Includes audios and videos of conference presenters.

NOTE: Dr. Bernard Bihari's friend and colleague, Dr. Gluck is a committed LDN advocate. He contributed a chapter to *Honest Medicine*.

LDN Research Trust

https://www.ldnresearchtrust.org

Linda Elsegood's very extensive LDN website. Contains a great deal of information about LDN, as well as links to Linda's more than 700 audio and video interviews with doctors, patients and compounding pharmacists who share their experiences of prescribing, compounding and using LDN. Lists LDN websites, Facebook groups, and forums throughout the world. A wealth of information.

LDNScience.org

https://www.ldnscience.org

Considered a "physicians' LDN site." Created by research scientist Moshe Rogosnitzky, this site contains information about prescribing doctors and compounding pharmacists, as well as all the LDN studies to date. On a controversial note, the "LDN Science" site also lists a company that sells LDN to patients without a prescription. Most experts advise against this.

Crystal Nason

http://crystalangel6267.webs.com

Crystal is the multiple sclerosis patient and LDN advocate who curates the most extensive list of doctors who prescribe LDN throughout the world. While she does not list the names of the doctors on her site, patients are invited to email her, and she will send them the names and contact information for prescribing doctors in their states or countries. Her website contains compounding pharmacists by state, and lots of information about multiple sclerosis.

John Donnelly's LDNDatabase.com

http://www.ldndatabase.com

While this site/database is out of date, I am including it anyway, because it contains valuable information about individual patients' experiences taking LDN. The experiences are divided by condition. John's wife was a cancer patient. Although she has died, she and John both considered LDN to be a most valuable treatment.

LDN WEBSITES FROM AROUND THE WORLD

Thanks, in great part, to Linda Elsegood, LDN Research Trust, for these links. This list is constantly growing. See https://www.ldnresearchtrust.org/LDN_Websites

Finland, Maija Haavisto's Page

http://www.fiikus.net/?ldn

One of the contributors to this book, Maija is one of the foremost writers/researchers about treatments for chronic fatigue syndrome. A strong advocate for LDN.

LDN Italia

http://www.ldnitalia.org

The Italian LDN website was created by Emiliano Marchi, one of the contributors to this book. Emiliano also created and administers the Italian LDN Facebook group. The site lists pharmacies in Italy that compound LDN.

LDN Norway

https://sites.google.com/view/ldnno/startside

The Norwegian LDN website was created by Steinar Hauge, the LDN advocate who figures prominently in Frank Melhus's chapter in this book.

LDN for Autism / Dr. Brian Udell

http://www.theautismdoctor.com/low-dose-naltrexone-for-autism

Dr. Phil Boyle / Ireland

https://www.neofertility.ie

Dr. Boyle uses LDN in his medical practice in Ireland as part of his treatment for infertility. He has spoken at LDN conferences.

Africa: LDN and AIDS

http://ldnafricaaids.org

Bulgaria

http://www.alphamedica.eu

Germany

http://www.ldnhilft.org/

~

FACEBOOK GROUPS

These groups are often "members only" groups. In some cases, if you are not a member, you can still see information about the group when you access the link. In other cases, you will have to join first.

General Facebook Groups

LDN Got Endorphins?

https://www.facebook.com/groups/GotEndorphins

This group was started (and is administered) by Renée Foster, who has contributed her story to this book.

LDN Research Trust

https://www.facebook.com/groups/LDNRT

Linda Elsegood's group. Linda is one of this book's LDN Heroes.

Overcoming Autoimmune Disease with LDN

https://www.facebook.com/Overcoming-Autoimmune-Dis-eases-With-LDN-low-dose-naltrexone-250257402310

Low Dose Naltrexone (People Powered Medicine)

https://www.facebook.com/lowdosenaltrexone

LDN: A Journey to Health

https://www.facebook.com/groups/162953643802938

LDN Newbies Discussion Group

https://www.facebook.com/LDN-Newbies-Discussion-Group-179671852042942

LDN (Public Group)

https://www.facebook.com/groups/41763649443

LDN Users Chit Chat Group

https://www.facebook.com/groups/168458790027420

Disease- or Interest-Specific Facebook Groups

ME/CFS—LDN Low Dose Naltrexone ME/CFS Myalgic Encephalomyelitis/Chronic Fatigue

https://www.facebook.com/groups/200010163370187

Rheumatoid Arthritis—LDN for Rheumatoid Arthritis Disease (RAD)

https://www.facebook.com/groups/LDNforRAD

Hashimoto's—Low Dose Naltrexone (LDN) and Hashimoto's

https://www.facebook.com/groups/LDN4Hashi

Irritable Bowel Disease—IBD and LDN Chat Group
https://www.facebook.com/groups/IBDLDN/

Autoimmune Diseases—Overcoming Autoimmune Diseases with LDN (Low Dose Naltrexone)
https://www.facebook.com/Overcoming-Autoimmune-Dis-eases-With-LDN-low-dose-naltrexone-250257402310/

Thyroid Disease—Beating Thyroid Disease with LDN
https://www.facebook.com/groups/LDNthyroid

Chronic Illness and Infections—Low Dose Naltrexone (LDN) for Chronic Illness & Infections
https://www.facebook.com/groups/108424385861883

Alopecia—Treating Alopecia with Natural Healing and LDN
https://www.facebook.com/groups/143543962732869

Autism—Low Dose Naltrexone for Autism, LDN for ASD
https://www.facebook.com/groups/1622423624740752

Cancer—LDN for Cancer
https://www.facebook.com/groups/LDNforCancer

Fibromyalgia—Fibromyalgia & LDN
https://www.facebook.com/groups/125683697583815

Fibromyalgia—LDN og fibromyalgi i DK
https://www.facebook.com/groups/580554822061553

Beating Multiple Sclerosis with LDN

https://www.facebook.com/Join-the-Cause-of-Beating-Multiple-Sclerosis-with-LDN-low-dose-naltrexone-78735454559

Pet Health—Love Our Pets: Low Dose Naltrexone (LDN)

https://www.facebook.com/groups/LOVEOURPETSLDN

Country-Specific Facebook Groups

France: LDN Français—Naltrexone à Faibles Doses

https://www.facebook.com/groups/529573720481287/

Germany: LDN Low-dose Naltrexon (Deutschland)

https://www.facebook.com/groups/315938001858805/

Netherlands: LDN Gebruikersgroep

https://www.facebook.com/groups/LDNgebruikersgroepNederland/

Norway: LDN Norge

https://www.facebook.com/groups/262889817077593

Norway: LDN Erfaringer i Norge

https://www.facebook.com/groups/LDNiNorge/

Italy: Gruppo LDN Italia

https://www.facebook.com/groups/189026731227/

Turkey: LDN Türkiye

https://www.facebook.com/groups/256049790729/

Canada: LDN Canada Group

https://www.facebook.com/groups/789994561028433

Finland: LDN Finland

https://www.facebook.com/groups/523605491021007

Poland: LDN (Low Dose Naltrexone) PL—Stosowanie, Informacje, Wymiana Doświadczeń

https://www.facebook.com/groups/LDN.Polska

OTHER LDN FORUMS, INCLUDING YAHOO GROUPS

Spotlight LDN for MS

https://groups.yahoo.com/neo/groups/spotlight_ldn/info

United Kingdom: LDN Now

http://ldnnow.com

German LDN Forum

http://www.ldn4ms.de

LDN Yahoo Support Forum

https://groups.yahoo.com/neo/groups/lowdosenaltrexone/info

Thyroid Patient Advocacy

http://www.tpauk.com/forum/#additional_info

German-language Yahoo Group

https://de.groups.yahoo.com/neo/groups/ldn-deutschland/info

LDN EZ Board

https://www.tapatalk.com/groups/ldnlowdosenaltrexone

Autism and LDN

https://groups.yahoo.com/neo/groups/Autism_LDN/info

Healing Parkinson's—Destiny Marquez's Yahoo Group

https://groups.yahoo.com/neo/groups/healingparkinsons/info—

LDN CONFERENCES: 2005-2008

The LDN conferences from 2005 through 2008 were convened by Dr. David Gluck (http://ldninfo.org/events.htm).

2005—First Annual LDN Conference, NY Academy of Sciences, New York, New York

http://ldninfo.org/conf2005.htm

June 11, 2005—Speakers included Dr. David Gluck, Dr. Maira Gironi, Linda Elsegood, Dr. Bob Lawrence, Dr. Skip Lenz, Larry Frieders, Victor Falah, Fritz Bell, etc. Topics included Crohn's disease, multiple sclerosis, and the first published LDN book by Mary Boyle Bradley (*Up the Creek with a Paddle*). The site contains many audios and videos of presenters and panels.

2006—Second Annual LDN Conference, National Library of Medicine, Bethesda, Maryland

http://ldninfo.org/conf2006.htm

April 7, 2006—Among the speakers: Dr. David Gluck; Dr. Jill Smith, who, with Dr. Ian Zagon, conducted the LDN trials for Crohn's disease at Penn State; Dr. Jacquelyn McCandless, who devoted her life to helping children with autism, and used LDN; Dr. Phil Boyle; Dr. Skip Lenz; and Dr. Pat Crowley. Topics included multiple sclerosis, autism, and HIV. The site contains audios and videos of the speakers.

2007—NCI Conference: Low Dose Opioid Blockers, Endorphins and Metenkephalins, "Promising Compounds for Unmet Medical Needs," Bethesda, Maryland

https://www.lowdosenaltrexone.org/NCI_Conference_Apr_2007.pdf

April 20, 2007—Speakers included Dr. Jeff Abrams, Dr. David Gluck, Dr. Jill Smith, Dr. Ian Zagon, Dr. John Hong, Dr. Nicholas Plotnikoff, Dr. Burton Berkson, Dr. Maira Gironi, and Dr. Filippo Martinelli Boneschi, Topics included Crohn's disease, pancreatic cancer, colitis, and B Cell Non-Hodgkins Lymphoma.

2007—Third Annual LDN Conference, "Breaking Down Barriers," Vanderbilt, Tennessee

http://ldninfo.org/conf2007.htm

October 20, 2007—Speakers included Dr. Jaquelyn McCandless, Dr. Tom Gilhooly, Dr. Brendan Quinn, Dr. Pat Crowley, Dr. Terry Grossman, Dr. Burt Berkson, Dr. Jill Smith, and Dr. David Gluck. Topics included Crohn's disease, renal cancer, multiple sclerosis, and autism. The site includes video clips and a slide show.

2008—Fourth Annual LDN Conference, "A Revolution in Research," USC Health Sciences, Los Angeles, CA

http://ldninfo.org/conf2008.htm

October 11, 2008—Speakers included Joseph Wouk, author of *Google LDN*, Dr. Burt Berkson, Dr. Tom Gilhooly, Dr. Skip Lenz, Dr. Aristo Vojdani, Dr. Jaquelyn McCandless, and Dr. David Gluck. Topics included HIV/AIDS, autism spectrum disorder, multiple sclerosis, and pancreatic cancer. The site includes video clips.

∽

LDN CONFERENCES: 2009-2019

These conferences were convened by—or conducted with the assistance of—Linda Elsegood of the LDN Research Trust.

2009 — First European LDN Conference, Glasgow, Scotland

http://www.ldnresearchtrust.org/sites/default/files/March_2009.pdf

Organized by Dr. Tom Gilhooly. Speakers included Dr. Gilhooly, Dr. Phil Boyle, Steve Bagnulo, and Prof. Bob Self. Topics included Parkinson's disease, endorphin deficiency, psoriasis, infertility, and cancer.

2010 — Second European LDN Conference, Glasgow, Scotland

https://www.news-medical.net/news/20100310/2010-European-LDN-Conference-LDN-can-be-used-as-effective-treatment-for-people-with-MS.aspx

Organized by Dr. Tom Gilhooly. Speakers included Dr. Gilhooly, Dr. Jarred Younger, Dr. Pat Crowley, Dr. Skip Lenz, Stephen Dickson, Zoe Kamen, and Maija Haavisto. Topics included multiple sclerosis, chronic fatigue syndrome and fibromyalgia, Crohn's disease, irritable bowel disease, Parkinson's disease, and autism.

2010 — LDN Conference, Birmingham, England

http://www.ldnresearchtrust.org/sites/default/files/May%202010.pdf

Speakers included Dr. Tom Gilhooly, Dr. Bob Lawrence, pharmacist Stephen Dickson, MS Nurse Elaine Bosley, Dr. Phil Boyle, Dr. Jacquelyn McCandless, and Maija Haavisto. Topics included multiple sclerosis, infertility, autism, chronic fatigue syndrome, and HIV/AIDS. LDN users also spoke about their experience using LDN for a range of conditions. You can view Maija Haavisto's photographs from the Birmingham conference online at http://www.fiikus.net/?bhamldn.

2011—LDN Conference, Dublin, Ireland

http://www.ldnresearchtrust.org/sites/default/files/July%20 Newsletter%202011.pdf

Organized by pharmacist Brendan Quinn. Presenters included Dr. Patrick Crowley, Dr. Skip Lenz, Dr. Phil Boyle, Dr. Tom Gilhooly, Donald Reid, John Donnelly, and Linda Elsegood. Topics included cancer, multiple sclerosis, fibromyalgia, and arthritis. Here is a link to videos of the presentations: https://www.youtube.com/results?search_query=ireland+2011+ldn

2013—LDN Conference, "Autoimmune and Immune-Modulated Conditions," Chicago, Illinois

https://www.ldnresearchtrust.org/content/ldn-2013-conference

Speakers included Dr. Burt Berkson, Dr. Deanna Wyndham, Dr. Jill Smith, Dr. Mark Shukhman, Dr. Pradeep Chopra, Dr. Tom Gilhooly, Dr. Patrick Crowley, Pharmacists Stephen Dickson and Mark Mandel, and Paul Battle PA-C. Topics included alpha-lipoic acid and Low Dose Naltrexone, allergies, bowel syndrome (IBS), psychiatric disorders, and chronic pain. Powerpoint presentations are included. You can watch the speakers' presentations here: https://vimeo.com/channels/1320260

2014—LDN Conference, Las Vegas, Nevada

https://www.ldnresearchtrust.org/content/ldn-2014-conference

Speakers included Dr. Michael Arata, Dr. Phil Boyle, Dr. Tom O'Bryan, Dr. Pradeep Chopra, Dr. Pat Crowley, Dr. Samyadev Datta, Dr. Kent Holtorf, Dr. Akbar Khan, Dr. Audrey Lev-Weissberg, Dr. Armin Schewarzbach, Dr. Mark Shukhman, Paul Battle, and Claudia Christian. Topics included LDN in psychiatry, Lyme disease, weight loss, cancer, chronic fatigue syndrome, thyroid dysfunction, pharmacology of LDN, fertility, Crohn's disease, and small intestinal bacterial overgrowth (SIBO). The conference review is also online at: http://www.ldnresearchtrust.org/sites/default/files/The_LDN_2014_AIIC_Conference_Review.pdf

2016 — LDN AIIC Conference, Orlando, Florida

http://ldn2016.com

Speakers included Pharmacist Mark Mandel, Dr. Akbar Khan, Dr. Leonard Weinstock, Dr. Armin Schwarzbach, Dr. Jarred Younger, Dr. Skip Lenz, Dr. Jill Cottel, Dr. Tom O'Bryan, Dr. Kent Holtorf, Prof. Angus Dalgleish, and Dr. Phil Boyle.

2017 — LDN AIIC Conference, Portland, Oregon

https://www.ldnresearchtrust.org/conference-2017

Speakers included Dr. Jill Cottel, Dr. Anthony Turel, Dr. Paul S. Anderson, Dr. Armin Schwarzbach, Dr. Kent Holtorf, Dr. Deanna Wyndham, Paul Battle, and Stephen Dickson. Topics included cancer, psychiatry and psychotherapy, attention deficit and autism spectrum disorders, food-related disorders, Lyme disease, post-traumatic stress disorder (PTSD), and fibromyalgia. Livestream recordings of all the presentations are available for $40 to the public and $80 to medical professionals. The conference brochure is online at: https://www.ldnresearchtrust.org/sites/default/files/LDN%202017%20Brochure_1.pdf

2018 — LDN AIIC Conference, Glasgow, Scotland

https://www.ldnresearchtrust.org/conference-2018

Speakers included Dr. Stephen Dickson, Dr. John Kim, Dr. Richard Nahas, Dr. Julian Kenyon, Dr. Harpal Bains, Dr. Mark Cooper, pharmacist John Bardsley, Dr. Kent Holtorf, and Dr. Leonard Weinstock. Topics include cancer, multiple sclerosis, thyroid and hormone dysfunction, and intestinal conditions.

2019 — LDN Conference, Oregon

https://www.ldnresearchtrust.org/ldn-conferences

The conference is scheduled for June 7-9, 2019. Speakers and topics are being finalized as this book goes to press.

AUDIOS AND VIDEOS

There are hundreds of audios and videos about LDN throughout the Internet.

On all of the above conference websites, Dr. Gluck's conferences include audios and videos of all the speakers. Linda Elsegood's conferences include links to the presentations of all the speakers. Ms. Elsegood also offers streaming videos of ALL the presentations at her conferences for a very reasonable, nominal price.

Linda Elsegood has interviewed hundreds of people about their use of LDN: doctors, patients, compounding pharmacists.

LDN Video Interviews

https://www.ldnresearchtrust.org/ldn-videos

There is a drop-down menu to find interviews by topic/disease

The LDN Research Trust's VIMEO channel

https://vimeo.com/channels/ldnresearchtrust

Contains nearly 700 interviews so far. More are added every week.

LDN Radio Station

https://www.ldnresearchtrust.org/ldn-radio-station

BOOKS ABOUT LDN

The LDN Book—Linda Elsegood

https://www.amazon.com/LDN-Book-Little-Known-Naltrexone-Revolutionize/dp/1603586644

Honest Medicine: Effective, Time-Tested, Inexpensive Treatments for Life-Threatening Diseases — Julia Schopick

https://www.amazon.com/Honest-Medicine-Time-Tested-Inexpensive-Life-Threatening/dp/0982969007

Up the Creek with a Paddle — Mary Boyle Bradley

https://www.amazon.com/Creek-Paddle-Autoimmune-Disorders-Naltrexone/dp/1432711504

LDN for Parkinson's Disease — Robert Rodgers, PhD and Lexie Lindstrom

https://www.amazon.com/LDN-Parkinsons-Disease-Dose-Naltrexone/dp/1495924408

Promise of Low Dose Naltrexone Therapy: Potential Benefits in Cancer, Autoimmune, Neurological and Infectious Disorders — Elaine Moore and SJ Wilkinson

https://www.amazon.com/Promise-Low-Dose-Naltrexone-Therapy/dp/0786437154

Low Dose Naltrexone (LDN) Therapy: An Evidence-Based Review and Case Histories — Kim and Ely

https://www.amazon.com/Low-Dose-Naltrexone-LDN-Therapy/dp/1977098487

Google LDN — Joseph Wouk

https://www.amazon.com/Google-LDN-Joseph-Wouk/dp/0578004399

Talking Back to MS: How I Beat Multiple Sclerosis Using Low-Dose Naltrexone — Elizabeth Rhodes

https://www.amazon.com/Talking-Back-MS SclerosisNaltrexone/dp/1482605945/

LDN: Niedrig dosiertes Naltrexon – eine vielversprechende Therapie bei MS, Morbus Crohn, HIV, Krebs, Autismus, CFS und anderen Autoimmun- und neurodegenerativen Erkrankungen—Josef Pies (Autor) [Broschiert] (German-language LDN book)

https://www.amazon.com/LDN-vielversprechende-Autoimmun-neurodegenerativen-Erkrankungen/dp/B00FBBT3YM

BOOKS THAT CONTAIN INFORMATION ABOUT LDN

Hashimoto's Thyroiditis: Lifestyle Interventions for Finding and Treating the Root Cause—Izabella Wentz

https://www.amazon.com/Hashimotos-Thyroiditis-Lifestyle-Interventions-Treating/dp/0615825796

Scary Diagnosis: How I Took Charge Of My Health and Life and How You Can Take Charge of Yours—Alan Geller

https://www.amazon.com/Scary-Diagnosis-Charge-Health-Yours/dp/0978274806_

Children with Starving Brains: A Medical Treatment Guide for Autism Spectrum Disorder—Dr. Jaquelyn McCandless

https://www.amazon.com/Children-Starving-Brains-Treatment-Spectrum/dp/1883647177

Good News for People with Bad News—Nyema Hermiston

https://www.amazon.com/Good-News-People-Bad/dp/1504300653/ref=asap_bc?ie=UTF8

Fighting the Dragon: How I Beat Multiple Sclerosis — Sandra Kischuk

https://www.amazon.com/Fighting-Dragon-Beat-Multiple-Sclerosis/dp/1481025325_

Melissa vs. Fibromyalgia: My Journey Fighting Chronic Pain, Chronic Fatigue and Insomnia — Melissa Reynolds

https://www.amazon.com/Melissa-Fibromyalgia-Journey-Fighting-Insomnia/dp/1973384256

LDN DOCUMENTARIES

"The LDN Story"
Produced by Linda Elsegood, LDN Research Trust
https://vimeo.com/131314110

"LDN and Cancer: A Game Changer"
Produced by Linda Elsegood, the LDN Research Trust
https://vimeo.com/168562089

"Lyme Disease"
Produced by Linda Elsegood, LDN Research Trust
https://www.ldnresearchtrust.org/ldn-lyme-disease

Norwegian LDN Documentary
Created/produced by Frank Melhus, Producer at TV2 in Norway, one of the contributors to this book
https://www.youtube.com/watch?v=MChB37N9bF0

LDN PRESCRIBING DOCTORS

Doctors who prescribe LDN usually do not want to be listed publicly, probably because they are afraid of retribution from their fellow doctors. However, any patient who wants to find a doctor to prescribe LDN can do so in one of the following ways.

First, two websites offer names and contact information of doctors who have agreed to have their names and contact information listed publicly. They include:

LDN Prescribers List, from Linda Elsegood, LDN Research Trust

https://www.ldnresearchtrust.org/

LDN Science "Find a Doctor"

https://www.ldnscience.org/patients/find-a-doctor

Crystal Nason

You can also contact Crystal Nason, who has compiled a list of prescribing doctors in the US and abroad. She also has a list of doctors who will prescribe LDN over the phone. You can email her at angelindisguiseldn@yahoo.com. She will send you the names and contact information for doctors in your particular state.

COMPOUNDING PHARMACIES

Compounding pharmacists are listed in several places:

Dr. Gluck's Websites: LDNInfo.org and LowDoseNaltrexone.org

http://ldninfo.org/#How_can_I_obtain_LDN

LDN Science Website

https://www.ldnscience.org/patients/where-to-buy-ldn

Crystal Nason's Website

http://crystalangel6267.webs.com/ldn-compounding-pharmacies

LDN STUDIES

LDN studies are being conducted all the time. Here are some of the best known.

Crohn's Disease

Three studies at Penn State, conducted by Ian Zagon, PhD, and Jill Smith, MD.

"Low-dose naltrexone therapy improves active Crohn's disease." Published by the *American Journal of Gastroenterology*, 2007 Apr;102(4):820-8. Epub 2007 Jan 11. http://www.ncbi.nlm.nih.gov/pubmed/17222320

"Therapy with the Opioid Antagonist Naltrexone Promotes Mucosal Healing in Active Crohn's Disease: A Randomized Placebo-Controlled Trial" Published by *Digestive Disease Science*. 2011 Mar 8. http://www.ncbi.nlm.nih.gov/pubmed/21380937

"Safety and tolerability of low-dose naltrexone therapy in children with moderate to severe Crohn's disease: a pilot study." Published by the *Journal of Clinical Gastroenterology*. 2013 April. http://www.ncbi.nlm.nih.gov/pubmed/23188075

Fibromyalgia

Three studies conducted by Jarred Younger, PhD, at Stanford.

"Fibromyalgia symptoms are reduced by low-dose naltrexone: a pilot study." Published in Pain Medicine, 2009 May-Jun;10(4):663-72. Epub 2009 Apr 22. http://www.ncbi.nlm.nih.gov/pubmed/19453963

"Low-dose naltrexone for the treatment of fibromyalgia: findings of a small, randomized, double-blind, placebo-controlled, counterbalanced, crossover trial assessing daily pain levels." Published in *Arthritis & Rheumatism*, 2013 Feb;65(2):529-38. https://www.ncbi.nlm.nih.gov/pubmed/23359310

"The use of low-dose naltrexone (LDN) as a novel anti-inflammatory treatment for chronic pain." Published in *Clinical Rheumatology*, 2014; 33(4): 451–459. Published online 2014 Feb 15. https://link.springer.com/article/10.1007/s10067-014-2517-2

Multiple Sclerosis

"Pilot trial of low-dose naltrexone and quality of life in multiple sclerosis." Bruce Cree, University of California/San Francisco. Published in the *Annals of Neurology*, 2010 Aug;68(2):145-50. http://www.ncbi.nlm.nih.gov/pubmed/20695007

"A pilot trial of low-dose naltrexone in primary progressive multiple sclerosis." Maira Gironi, MD, Milan, Italy. Published in *Multiple Sclerosis*, 2008 Sep;14(8):1076-83. http://www.ncbi.nlm.nih.gov/pubmed/18728058

Hailey-Hailey Disease

"Treatment of Hailey-Hailey Disease with Low-Dose Naltrexone." Published in *JAMA Dermatology* 2017, Oct 1;153(10):1018-1020. https://www.ncbi.nlm.nih.gov/pubmed/28768313

"Low-dose naltrexone: a novel treatment for Hailey-Hailey disease." Published in the *British Journal of Dermatology*, 2017 Oct 9. https://www.ncbi.nlm.nih.gov/pubmed/28991360

OTHER STUDIES AND TRIALS

Other studies and information about clinical trials are featured at these websites:

LDN Research Trust

https://www.ldnresearchtrust.org/ldn-clinical-trials

LDN Science "Clinical Trials in Progress"
https://www.ldnscience.org/patients/clinical-trials-in-progress

Low Dose Naltrexone (Trial Information)
http://www.lowdosenaltrexone.org/

POSTSCRIPT: UPDATE

In Chapter 10, a Hailey-Hailey disease patient describes how LDN helped heal her Hailey-Hailey disease (HHD). She also tells how the LDN/HHD case study that appeared in *JAMA Dermatology* made dermatologists aware of LDN as a viable treatment for this difficult-to-treat genetic skin condition.

After Chapter 10 was completed, patient advocate Cindy Siegel Shepler told me the fascinating story about how the study in *JAMA Dermatology* came about. I am including it here.

In 2014, the Hailey-Hailey Disease Worldwide Support Group approached the Rare Genomics Institute (https://www.raregenomics.org/), a platinum-rated non-profit organization dedicated to facilitating research opportunities on behalf of rare diseases. The HHDWSG collaborated with RG to help increase awareness of the use of LDN for HHD. To that end, in July 2016, RG published a review article summarizing the rationale for using LDN for HHD. The title: "Could Low-Dose Naltrexone be an Effective Treatment for Hailey-Hailey Disease?"*

https://www.raregenomics.org/blog/2016/9/11/could-low-dose-naltrexone-be-an-effective-treatment-for-hailey-hailey-disease

Following the publication of the article by RG in 2016, *JAMA Dermatology* published two case studies of three patients who were helped by LDN in October 2017, and one of the case studies in *JAMA Dermatology* cites the 2016 RG publication.

https://jamanetwork.com/journals/jamadermatology/article-abstract/2646785

https://jamanetwork.com/journals/jamadermatology/article-abstract/2646786

To my knowledge, this was the first instance of LDN being written about in a publication of the American Medical Association. LDN has, however, been featured in medical publications worldwide as a treatment for fibromyalgia, Crohn's disease, and MS—as well as for many other conditions.

https://www.ldnscience.org/research

*Note: While the original publication by RG from 2016 in *Molecular Medicine Letters* has been removed due to the cancellation of the journal, the publishing group, Gratis Open Access Publishers, has made the article available in another journal, *Integrative Biomedical Sciences* (http://www.gratisoa.org/journals/index.php/GJBS/article/view/1257/940). RG is currently working to have the publishers reflect the accurate publication dates and journal.

EASY ACCESS TO THIS BOOK'S HYPERLINKS

A word about Internet links in this book. *The Power of Honest Medicine* is full of resources, many listed as links to websites and PDFs. Due to the challenge of formatting electronic links in a printed book, you may find it difficult to access them. I am therefore providing a website which contains all the live links in this book, divided by chapter.

http://www.honestmedicine.com/TPOHMHyperlinks.html

APPENDIX B

ABOUT THE AUTHORS

Julia Schopick

Julia Schopick is the author of the best-selling book, *Honest Medicine: Effective, Time-Tested, Inexpensive Treatments for Life-Threatening Diseases.* She wrote *Honest Medicine* as a result of becoming an advocate for her husband, Tim Fisher, who was a 15-year survivor of a cancerous brain tumor, even though his doctors "gave him" a maximum of three years to live. Both she and Tim felt that his extra years of life were a result of Julia's unrelenting research for treatments to increase his survival and quality of life. Unfortunately, his doctors were not interested in learning about these treatments.

Julia decided that her mission was to teach patients about treatments like those she found for Tim through her writings and her online presence. Hence, *Honest Medicine* is about four science-based treatments most doctors don't know about and aren't interested in learning about.

One of the four treatments is Low Dose Naltrexone (LDN).

Julia is a seasoned radio guest who has appeared on over two hundred shows to promote her book. Over the years, she found that LDN was the most-asked-about treatment of the four, which is why she decided to write an entire book about it.

Through her writings, her "Honest Medicine" blog—located at http://www.HonestMedicine.com—and her presence on social media (especially Facebook), Julia has been realizing her goal of empowering patients to make the best health choices for themselves and their loved ones. She hopes to continue this mission for many years to come. You may reach her via email at Julia@HonestMedicine.com.

∽

Don Schwartz

Don Schwartz is an author, journalist, personal historian, and actor whose goal is to enhance the lives of people and non-human animals through his work. Since 1977, his writings have appeared in a variety of publications. His book, *Telling Their Own Stories: Conversations with Documentary Filmmakers* (2013), is available on Amazon in both print and ebook versions.

Since 2010, Don's more than 400 documentary reviews have appeared online in FromTheHeartProductions.com, *CineSource Magazine*, and *The Marin Post*. He has reviewed several documentaries that address shortcomings and solutions in the medical profession and industry.

Starting in 2002, Don has been utilizing his talents as a professional actor by working as a Standardized Patient, assisting in the training of healthcare professionals, both graduate and undergraduate—as well as practicing nurses and physicians. His work takes him throughout the San Francisco Bay Area. Don has worked with students from schools of medicine, nursing, physician's assistants, podiatry, and many other allied health care professions. Through these programs, he portrays patients with various illnesses so that medical professionals and professionals-in-training may become more empathetic and compassionate caregivers. Don considers this an essential part of his mission to make the world a better place.

Don holds a bachelor's degree in Psychology from Emory University, a Master's in Humanistic Psychology from the University of West Georgia, and a PhD in Integral Counseling and Psychotherapy from the California Institute of Integral Studies.

Learn more about his work at his website, http://www.DonSchwartzServices.com

Endnotes

Introduction

1 An off-label treatment is one that a physician prescribes for a condition other than the one or ones it was approved for by the FDA. Every doctor has the right to do this, but pharmaceutical companies are not allowed to promote a drug for off-label use.

2 http://www.honestmedicine.com/ldnteleseminar.html

3 http://www.honestmedicine.com/ldn-coaching.html

4 http://www.tv2.no/a/4037140

5 http://www.diabetesed.net/page/_files/autoimmune-diseases.pdf. The statistics provided in this 2011 *The Cost Burden of Autoimmune Disease: The Latest Front in the War on Healthcare Spending*, are the most recent. This is a joint publication of the American Autoimmune Related Diseases Association (AARDA) and the National Coalition of Autoimmune Patient Groups (NCAPG).

6 Dr. Bihari's original work with LDN was with AIDS patients: http://honestmedicine.typepad.com/ldn_teleseminar/Alternative-Therapies_Bihari-reprint.pdf

7 http://www.lowdosenaltrexone.org/index.htm#pharmlist

8 http://www.ncbi.nlm.nih.gov/pubmed/17222320

9 http://www.ncbi.nlm.nih.gov/pubmed/21380937

10 http://www.ncbi.nlm.nih.gov/pubmed/23188075

11 http://www.ncbi.nlm.nih.gov/pubmed/23359310

12 http://www.ncbi.nlm.nih.gov/pmc/articles/PMC3962576

13 http://www.ncbi.nlm.nih.gov/pubmed/19453963

14 http://www.ncbi.nlm.nih.gov/pubmed/20695007

15 https://www.ncbi.nlm.nih.gov/pubmed/18728058

16 https://www.ncbi.nlm.nih.gov/pubmed/28768313

17 https://www.ncbi.nlm.nih.gov/pubmed/28991360

18 http://www.lowdosenaltrexone.org/events.htm

19 http://www.ldnresearchtrust.org/ldn-conferences

20 http://www.lowdosenaltrexone.org

21 http://www.ldnresearchtrust.org

22 https://vimeo.com/channels/ldnresearchtrust

23 https://vimeo.com/ldnresearchtrust So far, there are nearly 700 interviews

on this site. The number is ever-growing.

24 http://www.ldnresearchtrust.org/LDN_Websites

25 http://www.honestmedicine.com/ldnteleseminar.html

26 http://www.honestmedicine.com/ldn-coaching.html

27 http://www.blogtalkradio.com/parkinsons-recovery/2011/10/05/low-dose-naltrexone

28 http://www.blogtalkradio.com/parkinsons-recovery/2014/02/05/low-dose-naltrexone-for-parkinsons

29 http://instantteleseminar.com/?eventID=53143554

30 http://instantteleseminar.com/?eventid=55729641

SECTION I: UNDERSTANDING LDN AND AUTOIMMUNITY

Chapter 1: The LDN Story

31 I want to thank Dr. Burt Berkson for introducing me to this quote. It is one of his favorites.

32 http://www.honestmedicine.com/2011/05/bihari-video.html. The transcription of this video of Dr. Bihari was reprinted with my permission in the March/April 2013 issue of *Alternative Therapies Magazine*.

33 He experimented with lower and lower doses and finally settled on 3 mg. Other researchers advocated for 4.5 mg, and Dr. Bihari eventually started prescribing it at that dose. In a recent interview, Dr. Lenz stated that Dr. Bihari was not initially receptive to the switch to 4.5 mg.

34 http://www.lowdosenaltrexone.org/gazorpa/interview.html

35 http://honestmedicine.typepad.com/ldn_teleseminar/Alternative-Therapics_Bihari-reprint.pdf

36 http://www.ldnresearchtrust.org/how-naltrexone-works

37 http://www.lowdosenaltrexone.org/index.htm#pharmlist This website also contains an excellent description of reliability problems with many compounding pharmacies that purport to compound LDN, and what to watch out for when choosing a compounder: http://www.lowdosenaltrexone.org/comp_pharm.htm

38 i.e., slowly weaning

39 Much of the interest in LDN in Norway is the result of the documentary produced by Frank Melhus for the Norwegian television station TV2. See http://www.tv2.no/a/4037140.

40 There are videos of many of these prescribing doctors on the LDN Research Trust's Vimeo channel, https://vimeo.com/channels/ldnresearchtrust, as well as at the LDN conferences, http://www.lowdosenaltrexone.org/events.htm.

Chapter 2: Autoimmune Diseases

41 A medical writer and author of women's fiction, over the years Virginia has served as a co-author and ghostwriter for several books on medical topics, including, with Paul Harch, MD, *The Oxygen Revolution: Hyperbaric Oxygen Therapy (HBOT): The Definitive Treatment of Traumatic Brain Injury (TBI) & Other Disorders.*

42 http://www.autoimmunemom.com/new-autoimmune-start-here/12-super-symptoms.html

43 This statistic also appears in a publication from 2011; it is invariably an underestimate even today.

44 http://hub.jhu.edu/gazette/2014/july-august/what-ive-learned-noel-rose/ — an interview with Dr. Rose, conducted in 2014. He is often referred to as the "father of autoimmunology."

45 https://www.amazon.com/Autoimmune-Epidemic-Donna-Jackson-Nakazawa/dp/0743277767

46 http://www.hopkinsmedicine.org/news/publications/johns_hopkins_health/fall_2013/winning_the_battle_within

47 http://www.diabetesed.net/page/_files/autoimmune-diseases.pdf. The statistics provided in this 2011 publication are the most recent.

48 http://www.honestmedicine.com/2011/05/bihari-video.html

49 The interview was reprinted by *Alternative Therapies Magazine* in their March/April 2013 issue: http://honestmedicine.typepad.com/ldn_teleseminar/Alternative-Therapies_Bihari-reprint.pdf

50 https://www.youtube.com/watch?v=Z9pRy8lJxHs

51 https://www.ldnresearchtrust.org/conditions

52 https://www.amazon.com/Living-Well-Autoimmune-Disease-You-That/dp/0060938196/. Ms. Shomon also has disease website, http://www.mary-shomon.com and Facebook group, http://www.facebook.com/ThyroidSupport

53 http://americannewsreport.com/nationalpainreport/miss-understood-fibromyalgia-ignorance-hurts-8823115.html

54 https://www.aarda.org/autoimmune-information/autoimmune-disease-in-women

SECTION II: THE LDN HEROES

Chapter 6: How Suffering Turned Linda Elsegood into an LDN Hero: A Tribute to Persistence

55 https://www.gov.uk/government/organisations/charity-commission/about

56 At last count, there are 240 conditions LDN might be able to help. https://www.ldnresearchtrust.org/conditions

57 https://vimeo.com/259613972

58 https://vimeo.com/131314110

59 https://vimeo.com/168562089

60 https://www.amazon.com/LDN-Book-Little-Known-Naltrexone-Revolutionize/dp/1603586644

61 https://www.ldnresearchtrust.org/sites/default/files/MyLDN_Health_Tracker_App.pdf

62 https://www.ldnresearchtrust.org/volunteering

63 https://www.ldnresearchtrust.org/donate

SECTION III: THE STORIES

Introduction

64 Please see this link from LDNResearchTrust.org: https://www.ldnresearchtrust.org/conditions

Chapter 7: Lad Jelen, Crohn's Disease

65 https://www.fistulafoundation.org/what-is-fistula/

66 Please see the author's note at the end of this chapter, for Dr. Jill Smith's comments. Dr. Smith is the physician who ran the trial Lad participated in.

67 Irritable Bowel Disease

Chapter 8: Maija Haavisto, Finland, Chronic Fatigue Syndrome/Myalgic Encephalomyelitis

68 http://www.epilepsy.com/learn/types-seizures/absence-seizures
69 http://cfs.gehennom.org/foorumi
70 http://cfs.gehennom.org/?kirja
71 http://www.brokenmarionettebook.com
72 https://www.facebook.com/groups/108424385861883
73 http://forums.phoenixrising.me/index.php?threads/olli-polo-finland-in-trouble-for-treating-pwme.54068
74 http://www.ilmestykset.net/in-english
75 http://www.hankalapotilas.net/in-english

Chapter 9: John O'Connell, Hashimoto's Thyroiditis

76 https://www.youtube.com/watch?v=QHTfy94mA5s
77 https://www.youtube.com/watch?v=OEiNjAcL12M
78 https://www.amazon.com/Google-LDN-Joseph-Wouk/dp/0578004399
79 https://www.amazon.com/Creek-Paddle-Autoimmune-Disorders-Naltrexone/dp/1432711504
80 https://www.amazon.com/Promise-Low-Dose-Naltrexone-Therapy/dp/0786437154
81 http://www.lowdosenaltrexone.org/gazorpa/interview.html
82 http://honestmedicine.typepad.com/ldn_teleseminar/Alternative-Therapies_Bihari-reprint.pdf

Chapter 10: May-Britt Hansen, Netherlands, Hailey-Hailey Disease

83 *JAMA*, the *Journal of the American Medical Association*, published by the AMA, is one of the best known of the journals read by physicians. There are *JAMA* journals for several specialties, including cardiology, dermatology, facial plastic surgery, internal medicine, neurology, oncology, ophthalmology, otolaryngology, pediatrics, psychiatry, and surgery.

Chapter 13: Lexie Lindstrom, Parkinson's Disease

84 http://www.blogtalkradio.com/parkinsons-recovery/2011/10/05/low-dose-naltrexone

85 http://mailtribune.com/archive/old-drug-new-use-

86 http://www.blogtalkradio.com/parkinsons-recovery/2011/10/05/low-dose-naltrexone

87 http://www.blogtalkradio.com/parkinsons-recovery/2014/02/05/low-dose-naltrexone-for-parkinsons

88 http://instantteleseminar.com/?eventID=53143554

89 http://instantteleseminar.com/?eventid=55729641

Chapter 14: Maureen Mirand, Rheumatoid Arthritis

90 http://articles.mercola.com/sites/articles/archive/2011/09/19/one-of-the-rare-drugs-that-actually-helps-your-body-to-heal-itself.aspx

91 http://www.lowdosenaltrexone.org

Chapter 18: Darlene Nichols, Lupus and Myasthenia Gravis

92 http://www.burzynskipatientgroup.org/antineoplastons

Made in the USA
Middletown, DE
01 April 2024